Conquer Stress *with* Grete Waitz

Best wishes to Susan

from

Grete Waitz

Conquer Stress

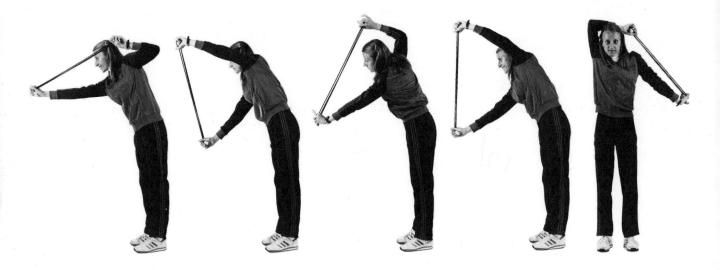

with Grete Waitz

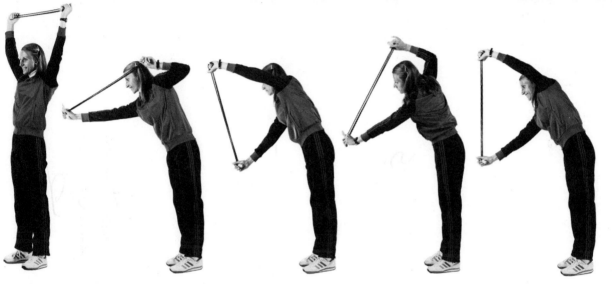

Grete Waitz,
Sigmund Strømme, and
Willi S. Railo

VNR VAN NOSTRAND REINHOLD COMPANY
NEW YORK CINCINNATI TORONTO LONDON MELBOURNE

Library of Congress Catalog Card Number 82-15929
ISBN 0-442-29243-0

Printed in the United States of America
Designed by Karin Batten
Photos by Tom Arma
Special thanks to Martina D'Alton
Illustrations on pages 99 and 108 by Sturla Kaasa

Published by Van Nostrand Reinhold Company Inc.
135 West 50th Street
New York, New York 10020

Fleet Publishers
1410 Birchmount Road
Scarborough, Ontario M1P 2E7, Canada

Van Nostrand Reinhold
480 Latrobe Street
Melbourne, Victoria 3000, Australia

Van Nostrand Reinhold Company Limited
Molly Millars Lane
Wokingham, Berkshire, England RG11 2PY

16 15 14 13 12 11 10 9 8 7 6 5 4 3 2 1

Library of Congress Cataloging in Publication Data

Waitz, Grete, 1953–
  Conquer stress with Grete Waitz.

  Translation of: Stress ned kom i form.
  Bibliography: p.
  Includes index.
  1. Stress (Psychology)   2. Physical fitness.
3. Physical education and training.   4. Substance abuse.
I. Strømme, Sigmund B., 1933–   II. Railo, Willi S.,
1941–   III. Title.
BF575.S75W3413   1983   158'.1   82-15929
ISBN 0-442-29243-0

Contents

	Preface	vii
1	The Stress in Your Life	1
2	The Program: Coping with Stress	5
3	Know Yourself: Self-Analysis at a Glance	25
4	Reading Your Mind: The Mental Symptoms of Stress	35
5	The Body's Message: The Physical Symptoms of Stress	45
6	Finding the Causes of Stress	66
7	The Keys to Better Health	80
8	Life Is Movement: Training for Your Health	90
9	Training for Competition	113
	Selected Reading	132
	Index	134

Preface

Amidst the rush of modern life, it has become increasingly difficult to find fulfillment and to build reserves of energy. In this book, we have addressed this problem and formulated a program to help most people cope with and overcome stress. Well-being and vitality are determined by closely related and equally important mental and physical factors. The program shows you how to use your own initiative and resources not only to rid yourself of stress, but to improve your life-style, get in shape, and thus regain vitality and a sense of well-being.

The training technique is based on the power of concentration. You will be shown a method for directing your mind to control your reactions to stressful circumstances. By thinking constructively, you will, in many cases, be able to reduce or avoid stress altogether. Mental training, however, is only a part of the book. You will also learn that the keys to health lie in a balanced program of mental training, regular physical activity, good diet, and adequate rest. The program has been tailored to help you avoid or control certain high-risk factors: the use and abuse of alcohol and drugs, the harmful smoking habit, excessive weight, high blood pressure.

Health has been defined as "the will to be healthy." Although this is a simplistic statement and, of course, much more is involved, in the final analysis good health is up to you. You must become actively involved to get the most out of this book. Go slowly, pause for reflection here and there, and look for applications to your unique problems. Remember too that there is a fine line of distinction between "normal daily stress" and the kind of psychological stress that requires professional and personal treatment. This book is not meant to take the place of such treatment. Nor will it cure every problem. It *will* suggest ways for solving your own problems.

The selection of topics and the method of presentation are based on our own experience and competence in our respective fields. We have also sought advice and expertise elsewhere, and are especially grateful to several of our colleagues who made very useful comments on the manuscript: Dr. Arne M. Benestad; Professor Per Lund-Johansen, MD; Dr. Helge Dyre Meen; and Dr. Lars Weiseth.

1 The Stress in Your Life

Damaging stress has become a fact of everyday life at one time or another for almost everyone. Debilitating stress-related diseases are increasing, and with them the need to control and eliminate stress overloads.

Yet it is completely normal to experience stress, and in some cases even necessary. The stress reaction is an alarm against danger, giving us a mechanism for survival. Primitive people, who were often exposed to danger, had precisely the same stress reaction that we have; it was an alarm system that enabled them to be constantly on guard, ready to defend themselves in the battle for survival.

Stress Reactions

With stress, a number of complicated physiological and psychological reactions take place within the organism. The heart begins to beat harder and faster, the muscles become tense, and breathing becomes quick and shallow. Some people become flushed; others begin to sweat. Stress even changes the biochemistry of the body, although relatively little is yet known about such change.

These reactions to stress are triggered by complex physiological mechanisms. Centers in the brain activate the sympathetic nervous system, leading to a secretion of the hormones adrenalin and nor-adrenalin, which in turn mobilize additional hormones. Among other

1

things, this prompts the release of sugar from the liver and a break-down of fat in the body's fat deposits, increasing the fat content of the blood. The blood pressure rises, and more blood is diverted from the gastrointestinal system to the muscles. There is also a tendency toward increased acid production in the stomach.

This physiological reaction to stress was especially useful for primitive humans in a "fight-or-flight" situation. Today, while such physical threats have been reduced to a minimum for most people, there remain many stress-related problems that elicit a fight-or-flight response in psychological terms. You become either aggressive or defensive. You choose either to take the offensive or to run away from the problem. Taking the offensive usually translates into constructive, problem-solving action. A defensive reaction—escape—usually means defeat, inactivity, lowered goals, and a loss of self-confidence.

To demonstrate this escape mechanism, we divided a number of people into two groups, telling them that they were to compete in solving simple mathematics problems. We chose three representatives from each group, selecting those who were looking down at their desks or shuffling papers around. We then told the groups that we had decided *not* to do the experiment after all, and we asked the following question: "Which of you were hoping not to be chosen?" In most groups, at least 80 percent admitted to having that hope. This is an example of a simple escape reaction. Most people try to get out of such a situation. Those who were chosen usually claimed not to be good at math and suggested that we choose someone else. Most people find similar "good" reasons for an escape reaction: "I'll do it later," "It's not really important anyway," "I don't have time." Another defensive reaction is to suppress the problem, refusing even to recognize that it exists.

How helpful, then, is stress in our society? For one thing, stress impulses, or what we sometimes call "demands," are necessary for human growth—both physical and mental. The human organism has a remarkable capacity to adapt itself to new situations and problems. For example, in order to develop strength, the muscles must be regularly exercised and given gradually increasing workloads. Similarly, to become psychologically strong, we must be exposed to a certain number of psychological demands. To develop a stronger will, we must put on the pressure from time to time. Parents who overprotect their children actually do them a disservice by not allowing them to experience problem-solving on their own. To become skilled at and capable of tackling difficult or demanding situations is a matter of practical training, of experiencing increasingly difficult demands.

A stress impulse also affects the brain's alertness. With little stress or stimulation, the brain is not very keen and we soon feel tired and listless. Under various types of stress, the brain's alertness level is raised and intensified, resulting in better concentration and a generally better capacity to work. Too many or strong stress impulses, however, will alarm the brain and reduce our ability to perform at capacity. This is especially so if the stress is caused by nervous anxiety, such as that which causes a simple mental block. Here, demand becomes overload.

The following questions are central in deciding whether or not stress is damaging your health: How often are you exposed to stress impulses? How strong is the stress impulse? How fast can you gear down following a stress impulse?

1. The frequency of stress impulses. The more often you are exposed to stressful situations the more likely you are to develop negative stress. Personality can play a major role in the development of negative stress. By now most readers are familiar with the Type A personality. This personality appears to have an enormous amount of energy, is active and aggressive, and angers at the drop of a hat. It is, for example, usually very impatient in such situations as traffic jams or waiting to be served in a restaurant.

    Ambitious and competitive, Type A personalities, seen superficially, appear to be decisive, energetic, and extremely self-confident. However, these people rarely take time for contemplation or self-reflection. They seek out one stress situation after another, forging ahead with clenched teeth until their health breaks down. They are their own worst enemies.

2. The intensity of stress impulses. It should be clear that the intensity of a stress impulse determines your stress reaction. Yet this intensity almost always depends on your interpretation of the stress-causing situation. A dramatic experience such as war, a catastrophe, an accident, or physical violence would be enough to create a relatively long-lasting stress reaction in almost anyone.

3. Gearing down after stress. A stress impulse takes you from a relaxed state to an anxious one. When the stress situation is over, you relax. How quickly you can relax is important; it is dangerous to take too long to return to a normal resting state, and some people do not return to this state at all. People who dwell on the stress impulse are usually slow to gear down. Such people are often chronic worriers with negative thoughts, who dread moving into the future and perhaps have a guilty conscience because they do not accomplish everything they should.

The faster you turn off the stress impulse, the sooner the stress situation is over and the sooner you relax.

The speed with which you return to the relaxed state depends on your general feeling of well-being. Fatigue makes gearing-down a difficult process. Studies have shown, for example, that after a vacation, industrial workers return more quickly to a relaxed state than before. In another study of stress reactions, subjects put in seventy hours overtime work over a four-week period. The most distinctive finding was an increase in stress reactions—in stress hormone levels, heart rate, irritability, and fatigue—when the subjects supposedly relaxed at home in the evening. The reactions were worse toward the end of the study even though work demands had not increased.

Such findings illustrate a kind of vicious circle that stress candidates often follow: stress impulses→negative stress reaction→less power of resistance against new stress impulses→new impulses produce more stress→more negative stress reactions occur more frequently→a further reduction in the power of resistance, and so on. As this pattern demonstrates, stress itself is not necessarily harmful, but your reactions to it can be.

In reading this chapter, you have taken the first step toward developing a constructive response to the problems of stress. Recognizing and understanding the stress in your own life is essential to making it work for and not against you.

2 The Program: Coping with Stress

The human brain is a fantastic instrument. It makes even the most advanced computer seem like the simplest of adding machines. Among other things, it allows you to change your life dramatically by helping you to reduce the level of stress in your life and develop yourself.

A few experiments will help to illustrate just how powerful your brain is when you concentrate. Stand with your back about five inches from a wall. Shut your eyes and repeat in your mind: "I am falling backward." Concentrate on the phrase. After a while you will notice that your body reacts to the message your mind is sending, and you will fall backward. Now turn around and face the wall. Again, close your eyes and this time repeat in your mind: "I am falling forward." Concentrate. Your body will soon respond and you may even touch the wall. There is nothing "mystical" about this, it merely demonstrates that your mental powers of concentration have a definite effect on the body.

Another simple experiment will demonstrate a psychological reaction that most people have experienced at one time or another. Before going to sleep, program yourself to wake up at a certain time: TOMORROW I WILL WAKE UP AT SIX O'CLOCK. Most people will obey the command and indeed wake up around six o'clock. You slept, but your subconscious did not.

These two small illustrations reveal the close relationship between your thoughts and reactions. Thoughts run through the brain in

Stand with your back five inches from a wall, close your eyes, and think, "I am falling backward."

Stand five inches in front of a wall, close your eyes, and think, "I am falling forward."

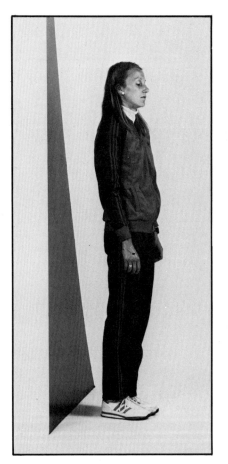 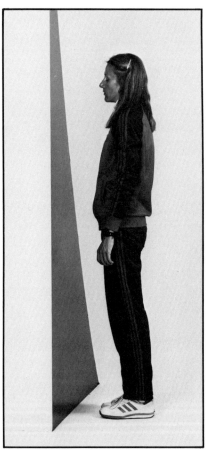

words, sentences, or images that describe what we see, hear, and experience. Two people will often have extremely different thoughts about a single phenomenon, and will also have different conscious and unconscious associations. Try another experiment. Shut your eyes and think for ten seconds about each of the following words: mother, success, nervous, fiasco, job. Notice the thoughts and feelings each word conjures up.

In your waking life, such conscious or unconscious mental processes are constant. The brain digests and processes information without always making a clear distinction between actual and imagined situations or events. The thinking process is similar in both cases. For example, when you told yourself that you were falling backward, you actually did. The body will react in the same way to other kinds of concentrated thoughts. Thus, the thought "I feel peaceful" will actually lead to a feeling of security. Such thoughts *precede* and to a large extent *control* feelings. This means that positive thoughts will normally lead to positive reactions in the same way that negative thoughts lead to negative reactions. To a large extent, your "inner conversations" determine what your psychological reactions will be. They also reinforce well-established roles and self-images: "I'm so stupid," "I'm so afraid," "I don't dare," "I'm shy." Obviously such statements only make matters worse. It would be better to say: "I'm clever," "I'm able to make decisions," "I can take the initiative," "I'm not afraid." Part of the training program in this book involves repeating such verbal exercises, called Training Sequences. Choose the best phrases for your own needs, but read through them all first, for you may become more aware of your own negative reactions. The exercises will help you to develop more positive inner conversations of your own.

Thus even though thought—which is a good weapon against stress—is inadequate in especially difficult situations when your basic psychological needs are left unsatisfied, you can use it to control and direct your behavior so that these needs are better fulfilled. In this way, you actively create more positive and constructive situations, instead of passively "letting things happen."

People often resist change, even for the better. Such resistance may mean that you are getting close to the core of your problems. As you read through this book, recognize the things you reject or find trivial, comical, or irritating. These may be signals to your problems. Other people turn new tasks into achievement tests and feel they must perform at top capacity. This type of reaction should be avoided, especially in connection with mental training. It leads only to a guilty conscience and increased stress.

THE PROGRAM.

The goal behind mental training is to help you to help yourself. This book will act as your instructor. The first week should be seen as a trial period in which you monitor your reactions to the training and allow your body to relax gradually. The beginner's program is so short that most people will not have achieved deep relaxation once it is finished. This will come later.

Stand easily, hands relaxed at the sides and shoulders down, and tip only your head to one side.

Let your head roll back. Do not strain.

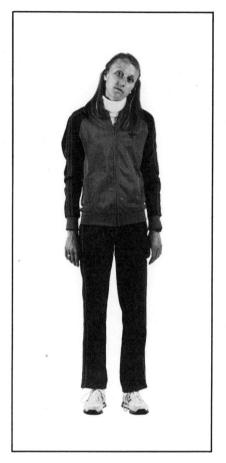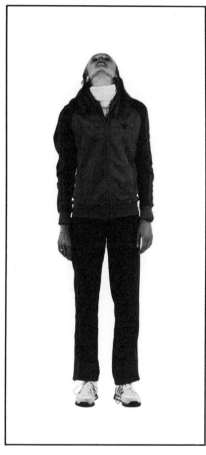

Step-by-Step

1. Preparation. It is important that you find a quiet place in which to train, and to be certain that you will not be interrupted during your thirty-minutes daily training period. You may even want to turn off the telephone during this time.

   If you already have a program of physical training—jogging, aerobic dancing, swimming, walking, bicycling—try to time it so that your mental training will immediately follow each exercise session. If you cannot arrange this, you should spend five or ten minutes doing gentle warm-up exercises, such as those shown here, before each mental training period.

2. The basic relaxation exercises. Sit in a comfortable chair or lie

Gently roll your head to the other side. Do not lift your shoulders, but let your ear lead toward the shoulder.

Roll your head forward toward chest. Feel the stretch at the back of your neck and let the weight of your head pull gently forward and down. Repeat this sequence five times, then reverse direction for five repetitions. Increase at your own pace.

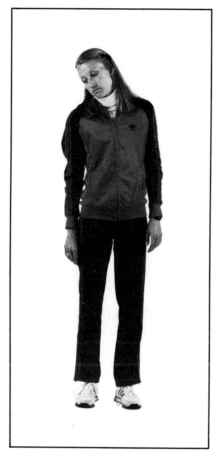
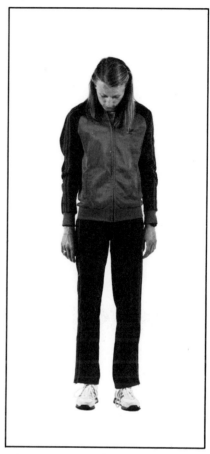

down on the floor on padding or a mat, or on a bed. It may also help to have quiet and relaxing music playing in the background.

Once you are settled and comfortable, close your eyes. Concentrate on your breathing. Regulate it so that it is slowly pulled deep down into your stomach, which should move in and out very slowly. Try to let the air go even deeper down, remaining calm and quiet as you breathe. If the sensation is pleasant, continue. If it is at all uncomfortable, stop at this point.

Begin to tense the muscles of your body, progressing downward from the face to the neck, chest, arms, abdomen, buttocks, legs, feet, and toes. Hold the tension to a count of five, then let go, allowing all your muscles to relax and become suffused with heat. You will feel the tension draining from each muscle as a relaxing warmth envelops them.

If the sensation is pleasant, continue to the next step, but if you experience any discomfort at this point, stop for the day.

Now once again tighten all your muscles, moving down the body from your face to your toes. Again hold the tension to a count of five and then let go, bathing your relaxed muscles in warmth. At the same time, concentrate on the following phrases:

BASIC TRAINING SEQUENCE #1

I am completely relaxed.
I am resting.
My stomach is breathing.
My breathing is deep and calm.

Repeat each exercise five to ten times. After about a minute, tense the muscles in your body and hold this tension for five seconds. If you have high blood pressure, tense your muscles only slightly. Then relax and move on to the next training sequence:

BASIC TRAINING SEQUENCE #2

My muscles are letting go of the tension.
My muscles are completely relaxed.
My muscles are resting.

Very soon you will begin to feel calm. Go back to the breathing exercise and repeat the Training Sequence. During the first week, spend only a few minutes a day on this training.

Standing easily, arms at your sides, scrunch your shoulders forward.

Rotate your shoulders up toward your ears without changing the position of your arms, neck, or head.

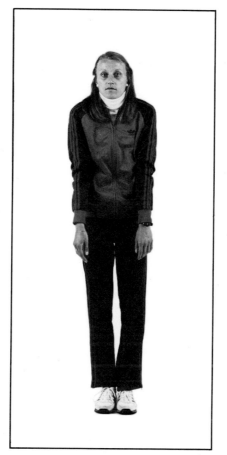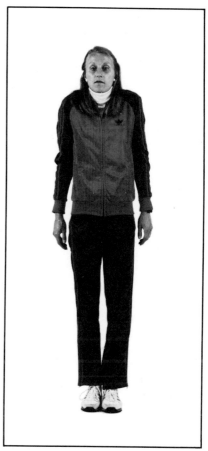

3. Advancing. If your reaction to these simple relaxation exercises is either positive or neutral, you may increase the training sessions to ten to fifteen minutes. If your reaction is negative, continue for only a few minutes until you feel ready to progress to a longer period.

4. Deep relaxation. After a week (or perhaps more) of practicing the initial Training Sequences for ten minutes or so, you should feel quite calm and relaxed. If not, continue to work twice a day through the routines. Do not rush ahead. But if you feel you have mastered the first steps, you are ready to start working on a deeper relaxation of the body. Begin with the warm-up exercises and the

Training Sequences in Step 2. When, after a few minutes, you begin to feel comfortably calm, you can again concentrate on your body. Give yourself plenty of time and begin from your head, moving down to your toes and using the following Training Sequence:

BASIC TRAINING SEQUENCE #3

My eyelids are relaxed.
My face is relaxed.
My tongue and jaw are relaxed.
My chin and cheeks are relaxed.
My neck is relaxed.
And so on with the *shoulders*, the *chest*, the *arms*, the *hands*, the *fingers*, the *stomach*, the *back*, the *buttocks*, the *upper thighs*, the *knees*, the *calves*, the *ankles*, the *toes*. After you have gone through your whole body, use the following awakening exercises:
I feel light and awake.
I feel awake and fresh.
I feel fresh and bright.

---

5. Concentration exercises: During the first three weeks of training you should be reading ahead, analyzing your own problems and determining which Training Sequences will be best for you. After three weeks spent exclusively on the basic exercises already described, you are ready to practice the concentration exercises in Training Sequences chosen from the book. Always begin with five to ten minutes of basic relaxation exercises, and do not use more than two to four of the Training Sequences during each session. Repeat each exercise of the sequence five to ten times before going on to a new one. Keep to the same sequence for about two weeks before adding or substituting a new one. You can also use these same exercises during your normal daily activities or when doing physical training.

In a fluid motion, rotate your shoulders backward. Do not change the position of your arms, but force your shoulderblades together.

Return to the starting position, arms hanging easily at your sides and shoulders squared. Now do the entire sequence in a fluid motion; do not jerk from one position to the next. Repeat ten times and increase at your own pace.

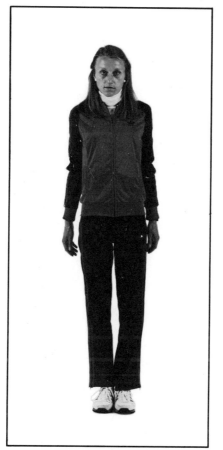
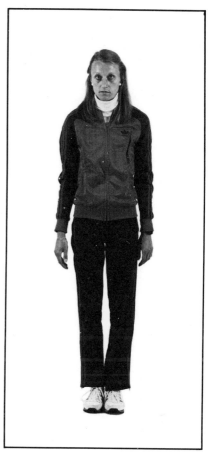

6. Applied training. When you have trained in the basic relaxation and concentration exercises for about two or three months and feel you have attained good relaxation, you can begin to work on concrete stress situations. For this step you will have prepared your own self-analysis sheet, as described in Chapter 3, and your own Training Sequences.

In your applied training, first do the relaxation exercises, both physical and mental. Once relaxed, imagine yourself in your own particular stress situation and work through the Training Sequence you have prepared or a suitable sequence from the book. The following basic sequence can be used in most situations:

With your legs together and arms extended to the side at shoulder height, make small circles with the full arm. Circle both forward and backward. Keep your hands extended and do not bend your elbows. Begin with ten counts in each direction and increase at your own pace.

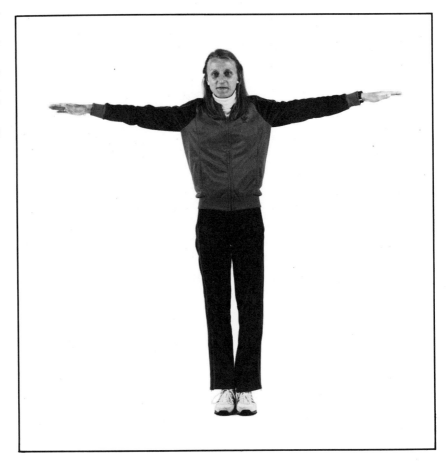

BASIC TRAINING SEQUENCE #4

I am completely calm.
I am completely relaxed.
I am calm and secure.
I can master the situation.
I have control over the situation.
I accept myself.
I feel strong and confident.

Stand with your legs comfortably apart, arms outstretched at shoulder level.

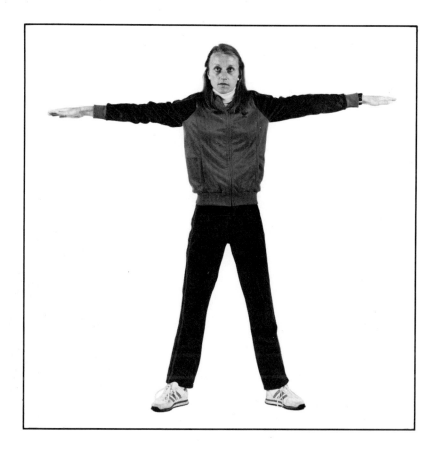

At first, do not work on more than one stress situation in each training session, and stay with the same situation for at least two weeks. Once you have better control of the different Training-Sequence methods, you can handle two or three stress situations in the same session.

REMINDERS AND SUGGESTIONS.

In the beginning, follow the Training Sequences in the order given and slowly repeat each phrase ten to fifteen times before going ahead. Do not work through the sequences frantically; deal with them systematically and calmly. No one expects anything special of you. Give

Touch the opposite toe with your outstretched hand, letting the other hand reach easily back and up. Do not strain, and do not force yourself to touch your toe; instead, reach only as far as you comfortably can, gradually increasing the stretch each time. Alternate sides and repeat twenty times in all. Increase at your own pace.

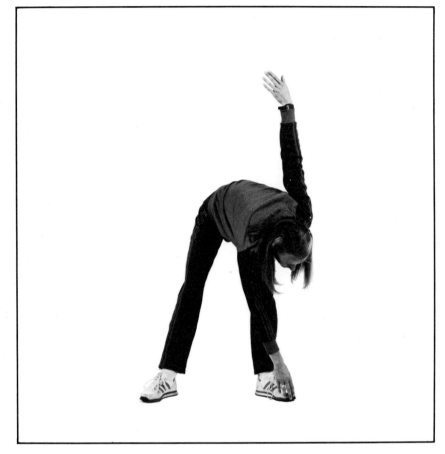

yourself the freedom and the time that you need, and do not turn your sessions into a competition. After a while it may be useful to alternate phrases and exercises so that your program includes both repetition and variation.

Train one or two times a day. It does not really matter *when* you train, but you should try to have fixed times, usually in the morning and again in the afternoon. You can even train in bed just before going to sleep. Once you are familiar with the techniques, you can take your training with you and work at it on the bus, at work, on the street, or when jogging.

Remember that all training takes time—including the exercise/re-

With your legs comfortably apart and arms on your hips with elbows bent, twist to the left. Keep both feet on the ground and twist only from your shoulders to your waist; do not let your hip follow.

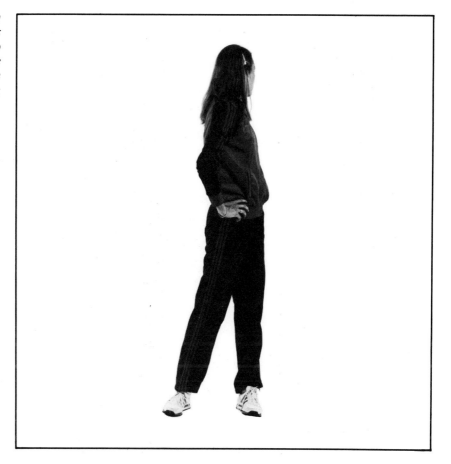

laxation type of training described here. Do not be impatient and do not expect immediate results. You should count on having relapses from time to time. Take breaks in the training if your motivation drops.

In the beginning, this type of training may be tiring. Some people may even find themselves falling asleep during training. However, this "beginner's reaction" will soon be replaced by a feeling of alertness and restfulness. Another common "beginner's reaction" is finding the initial results to be the opposite of those you had hoped to achieve. For example, a tension headache may actually become stronger at first. But as you continue, it will go away.

Return to center.

Now twist to the right. Continue to alternate twists for twenty repetitions. Increase at your own pace.

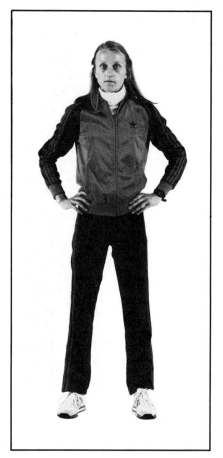
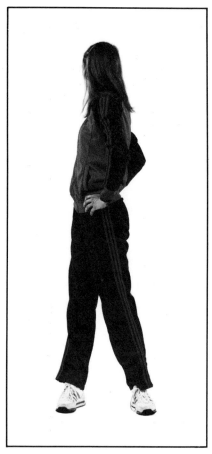

The beginner's program is designed to allow you to have constant control over and awareness of your own reactions. Some of these reactions may seem rather unusual or strange, but they are harmless. For example, as you train, parts of your body may begin to feel extremely heavy; or a tingling feeling may develop in your arms or legs; or you may begin feeling hot and sweaty. With time, such unusual reactions disappear.

For safety's sake, some people should consult their doctors before embarking on any new training program:

Those with very high or very low blood pressure who are already

While seated on the ground with your legs outstretched, toes flexed to the ceiling, and back straight, brace yourself lightly with your hands behind back. Inhale.

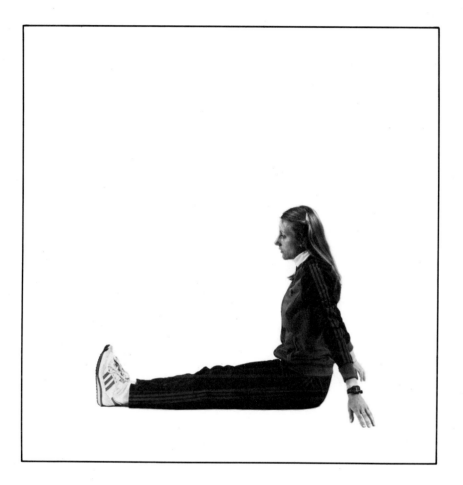

receiving medical treatment for their condition

Those with epilepsy

Those with a high level of anxiety needing anxiety-reducing medication

Those with heart problems

For monitoring your progress, isolating your problems, and jotting down the Training Sequences that best suit your needs, you should keep a journal. You will certainly need one for the self-analysis described in the next chapter. Also, once you've decided on a set of

On the exhale, reach forward to touch your toes. Do not strain farther than is comfortable; gradually increase the reach with each repetition, aiming for your toes. Use the exhale to move you farther toward your goal. Repeat ten times and increase at your own pace.

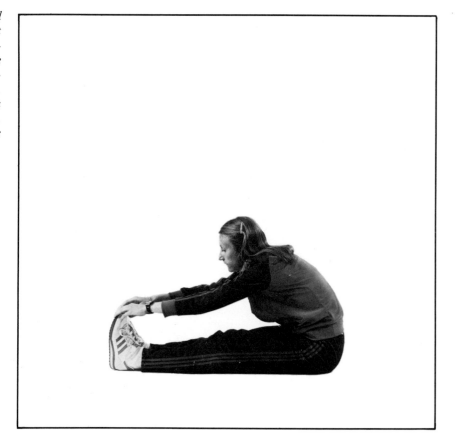

specific Training Sequences, even if only the four basic ones, you may find it helpful to make cassette tapes of them as a training aid. This will let you listen to and repeat the sequences while you train. If you do make tapes, be certain to speak clearly, slowly, and rhythmically, to include the proper number of repetitions of each phrase, and to leave several seconds of silence between each phrase.

BENEFITS.

It may increase your incentive to understand the main effects of mental training.

While lying on your back, bend your knees and fold your arms behind your head. Inhale.

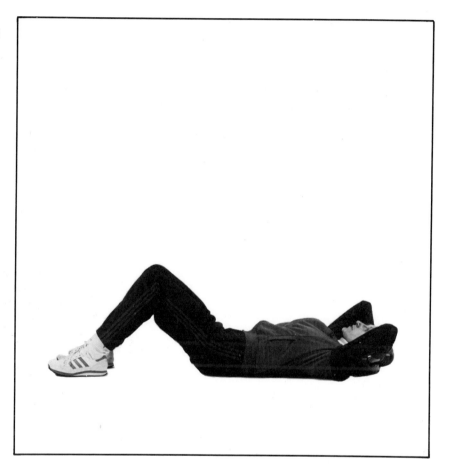

1. Relaxation and reduced stress. The autonomous nervous system usually functions by itself, regulating many important processes in the body, such as the beating of the heart or breathing. The relaxation program enables you to use your powers of concentration to partly control the autonomous nervous system and thus reduce the level of tension and stress in your life.

2. Increased ability to rest. Hard work and stress impulses often drain your energy and increase your need for rest and sleep. A state of deep relaxation can be an excellent supplement to sleep. Such relaxation will build up new reserves of energy after only a few minutes, and can be accomplished almost anywhere. And

As you exhale, lift your upper body with your abdominal muscles and touch your elbows to your knees. Do not lift with your back and do not strain. Repeat ten times; increase the number of repetitions at your own pace.

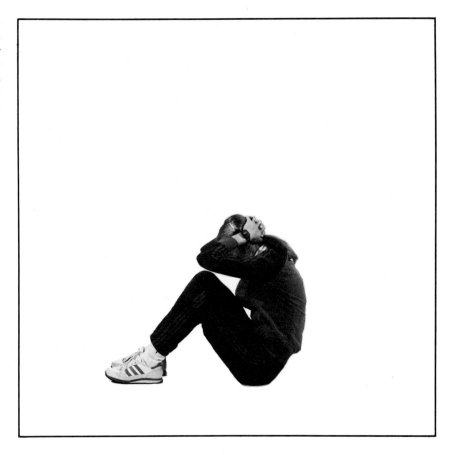

mental training can help overcome insomnia, as described in Chapter 5.

3. Increased ability to concentrate. A high level of tension often inhibits our ability to concentrate and to learn. In many cases, tension adversely affects the memory. Conversely, short daily periods of relaxation exercises will enhance your mental powers and enrich your creative experiences.

4. Self-awareness and self-analysis. Relaxation often leads to deeper self-knowledge. This is because you reach a high level of inner quiet and concentration, which is necessary for creative thought. At the same time, your defenses, which inhibit inner reflection, are gone.

Run in place while breathing freely. Lift your knees for greater exertion or maintain an easy jog. Try this exercise at first for thirty seconds and increase at your own pace.

Sit easily in a chair with your eyes closed. Breathe deeply from your abdomen.

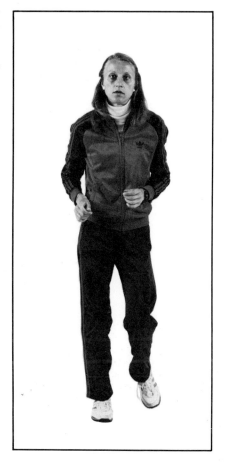

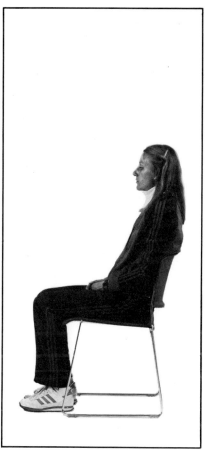

5. Problem solving. Stress-related problems will automatically be solved when you are more relaxed and in control of your nerves. However, other problems, directly related to concrete situations, may require more active work. This is especially true of problems caused by negative attitudes and reactions, or mental blocks. In all such cases, restructuring of the negative reaction to a more positive one is necessary, and the relaxation exercises and Training Sequences in this book will help you to isolate the problems and change your behavior patterns.

6. Changing destructive habits The mental training described here has helped many smokers to rid themselves of the habit. You can

Lie on a pad or mattress with your eyes closed. Breathe deeply from your abdomen.

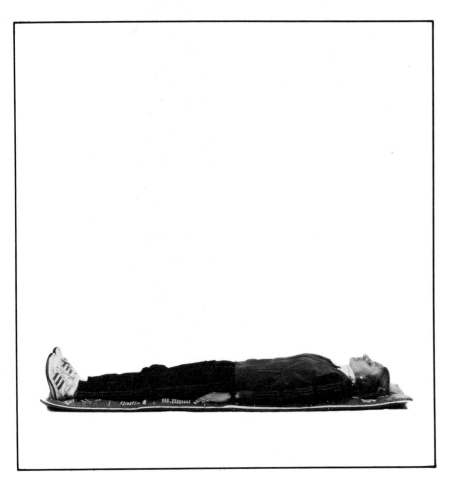

use the method to develop a negative attitude toward smoking and a positive one toward not smoking. The same technique is also very useful in dealing with milder forms of alcohol and drug abuse.

The basic mental training program and the four Training Sequences will be enough to help most people cope with a wide range of stress situations. By combining this training with an exercise program and following both programs regularly, you will be well on your way to reducing stress and channeling your energies into positive action.

3 Know Yourself: Self-Analysis at a Glance

Most people erroneously believe that they know themselves well. Try the following experiment: Give yourself three minutes to write down the four most positive aspects of your personality and the four most negative. Most people, if they answer truthfully, will find it hard to perform this simple task in the time allotted. Self-examination takes practice and is essential to positive self-development. But to the inexperienced it can be quite difficult, as the brief experiment demonstrates. When attempting to analyze yourself and discover your negative traits, you may become defensive; in fact, your defense mechanisms are automatically set in motion. It can be almost impossible to admit to mistakes. Instead you find a "good" explanation for your behavior. This can serve to reduce your anxiety and uphold your self-esteem, but can also easily fool you into thinking that you're something you are not, and further obscure your stress-related problems.

To try to figure out what you are like, read through the following section and carefully relate every point to yourself. Keep notes on your findings.

DEFENSE MECHANISMS.

When you are threatened, your defense mechanisms automatically take over. They either increase your feeling of self-esteem or decrease your level of anxiety and give you a more positive self-image. The illusions they create will prevent you from accepting certain realities. Study the typical defense mechanisms below.

1. Explaining our actions away. Some of the typical ways in which we excuse our actions are summed up in the following phrases.

   "I didn't like it anyway." This is a frequent psychological defense against defeat, frustration, or anxiety. Failure at work can be blamed on a dislike of co-workers or the job itself. "I don't care" is a variation on this, implying that with real interest you would have succeeded.

   "It's not my fault." Failure can also be blamed on someone or something in our environment: "I wasn't feeling well," "Everyone around me was so unreasonable," "They think only about themselves."

   "If I hadn't, no one else would have." As a psychological defense you may claim that your actions were necessary. An authoritarian leader can, for example, explain that "I had to make decisions since the others aren't mature enough to do so." Or a person who dominates the conversation may say, "I had to speak up or no one would have."

   "I'm not as bad as John is." Many defend their actions by comparing themselves to others and thereby feeling *relatively* good. You may say, for example, "I may be selfish, but John is even more selfish than I," or "I did a poor job, but Ellen's was even worse."

2. Identification. This means attributing other's positive qualities to yourself. Doing this conceals your own negative characteristics. For example, many husbands or wives will identify with their spouse's positive characteristics. Parents may identify with their children's successes or employees may identify with the cleverest of their fellow workers. Women especially will adopt their husband's status as their own.

3. Reverse reaction. Having a reverse reaction means covering up negative feelings by behaving in a contradictory manner. For example, the mother of an unwanted child may shower the child with attention; similarly, some people are particularly friendly with those they dislike.

4. Suppression. This psychological defense mechanism helps to systematically block out unpleasant memories. In some cases, people

are so clever at suppressing their problems that they end up forgetting about them completely; often what one calls forgetfulness is actually an active suppression of something unpleasant. But while suppression lets you push a problem aside, your reactions and behavior are usually affected by the problem.

5. Compensation. This means substituting a new activity for a weak one. Someone who is poor in academic studies may, for example, take up sports. Typically, those who compensate brag about their "good" characteristics and past achievements.

6. Humor. Making light of a problem is a classic defense mechanism. Yet it often gets to the point at which one takes *nothing* seriously. The distance between laughter and tears is often very short.

7. Withdrawal and Passivity. A simple defense mechanism is merely to withdraw into a state of passivity. In this state you avoid even what you may enjoy: meeting new people, going out, playing tennis, traveling, cultivating hobbies. Such withdrawal may give a sense of security, but in the long run it will only mean more stress.

SETTING GOALS.

Without goals, life becomes rather meaningless, boring, and dull. Yet the question of goals is not always whether or not you have them, but whether they are the right goals for you. Unrealistic goals cause stress. They may be too high or too many and insignificant for you.

1. Too-High Goals. If you are incapable of reaching your goals you will experience a feeling of failure or frustration. Even those who excel at what they do will experience this if their goals are too high. Today's world encourages you to set increasingly high goals, usually in the form of specific achievements; people are often judged *not* for what they are but for what they do or have accomplished. Yet with higher and higher goals you must work increasingly hard, and as a result you become stressed. Everyone needs challenges, but you must know your limits and your motives. In fact, setting increasingly high goals can become a *habit*. It is important to ask yourself: Is there always a good reason for fulfilling these goals? Is fulfillment worth the stress? Be aware of your own worth, no matter *what* your achievements. Your self-esteem should not depend

entirely on your accomplishments. Furthermore, many people strive madly to do what others expect of them. Keep in mind that it is often the expectations of parents, friends, colleagues, or spouses that define your goals.

Far too many people sacrifice their health and well-being in their race to achieve. And when the race is over, when they feel their goals have been reached, they may ask, "Have the battles and self-denial been worth it?" This is especially true of those who have developed stress diseases. The price was too high.

As long as you are happy in your efforts to reach your goals, you have no cause for concern. Set yourself reasonable and realistic goals that will not cost you your health, and remember that career and achievement goals are not the only goals in life.

2. Too many insignificant goals. A common cause of stress is the inability to differentiate between important and unimportant goals; equal effort is expended on achieving all goals: "I *must* advance in my job." "The house *must* always be neat." "I *must* be perfect." "I *must* not reveal any of my weaknesses." "I *must* have a new car." "I *must* win this argument." "I *must* earn more money." "I *must* always appear happy and friendly." "The children *must* do well at school." With this attitude you become just as frustrated over trivial as over important things.

When you recognize this pattern developing, stop and determine *which* goals are significant in your life and *why* they are. Do not just forge ahead at full speed, no matter how important a particular thing may be. And do not worry beforehand about whether or not a job will be well done, or feel insecure afterwards about your performance. If you do, your mind will become filled with small, insignificant worries, and you may destroy your health trying to sort them all out. Instead, take a bird's-eye view of your worries and, indeed, of yourself. It can be a very liberating experience.

"TEMPER, TEMPER."

Anger and irritation can both cause and result from stress. This is a normal reaction, but many people make life unpleasant for everyone around them with their bad moods. Some people seem to be constantly irritated about something, whether their job, traffic, spouse, children, or just life generally. Remember that irritation and aggression are *your* problems, and that while they can give you a feeling of power and importance, and can hide your failures, they often merely serve to lead you into conflict with other people. They indicate that you are incapable of solving a problem constructively.

Usually, you can defuse your anger by answering some simple questions: Is it out of proportion to its cause? Is there a better way of dealing with the problem? Are you using anger as a defense mechanism? Are you angry because you are insecure and do not accept yourself? Would you accept the same angry reaction in someone else? What problems does the anger solve?

YOUR SENSE OF HUMOR.

While some people resort to an extreme sense of humor as a defense mechanism, others lose it completely when under stress. Generally, it is advisable to keep a sense of humor. It does help to avoid stress-caused diseases, and makes it easier to see yourself from a distance in the situations you are in; dead seriousness has hardly ever helped anyone to recover from unhappiness.

You must recognize your behavior patterns in order to overcome the negative ones. Do you depend on strong defense mechanisms? Are your goals reasonable? Do you anger easily? Have you lost a sense of humor or a proper perspective on your problems? Can you even articulate the problem? Can you be open with yourself and finally accept yourself as you are?

POSITIVE THINKING.

To a great extent, your way of thinking decides how you experience things and what your reactions and feelings will be. It also determines whether or not you will be stressed.

No two people experience the same situation in the same way. Some feel stress while others may feel pleasure. Nearly every situation that you're exposed to in life has both positive and negative sides. But while negative thinkers typically dwell on earlier failures, positive thinkers emphasize their successes. They will also be much more optimistic about the future and, therefore, have fewer stress-causing worries. By finding the positive in all situations, and looking constructively at your experiences, you become better equipped to handle your difficulties.

Positive thinking is a habit that *can* be learned through experience. Unfortunately, so can negative thinking. Practice looking for the positive side of each new experience; in this way you will be able to think constructively and find solutions to problems when they arise. It is often possible to turn a "problem" into a positive situation, one that will enable you to grow as you solve it. Mental training helps you to form the habit of looking for and emphasizing the positive in every situation.

OPENNESS.

Problems or stress impulses usually grow until dealt with properly. In some cases, you may need to "live out" or experience the problem before it disappears. You will need to find outlets for tension and emotions. Bottling them up causes great stress. Mental training and physical exercise are excellent outlets. Being open about your problems and talking with others about them is also very helpful. Hiding your problems also causes stress and eventually may lead to an "explosion." You may have to force yourself at first to be a little more open. Talk to someone who is understanding and accepting and whom you feel you can trust.

ACCEPTANCE.

A common cause of stress is an inability to realistically accept ourselves and others. You may reproach yourself for not being what you or others expect you to be. Or you may feel that you have not lived up to your goals or potential. Many people who as children did not feel accepted by their parents have problems accepting themselves later in life. Learn to accept yourself by having a positive attitude toward yourself.

Many people are inflexible and intolerant, wanting others to be just like them and at the same time enjoying other people's faults. A kinder, more accepting attitude toward others is much more conducive to a nonstressful existence. It is better to try to change your own attitude than to try to change other people.

Seeking out situations in which you are accepted by other people not only increases your self-esteem but also reduces the stress in your life. Similarly, when you accept and help other people, you will usually find that others accept you in return. Be friendly and show interest in others. Give them the feeling that you respect and appreciate them. Be generous in praising and encouraging others. Criticize only if you can do it *constructively.* You should, however, also be aware of your own identity. Some people may overdo selflessness to the point at which they lose their own identity. They do not dare to oppose or resist other people's views—they *only* accept. Obviously this is going too far; there is a danger that such people will let others take advantage of them, which can lead to stress. Be aware of the subtle distinction between seeking acceptance and being used.

BACK TO BASICS.

There is a clear tendency in our society to value the more complicated things and neglect the simpler ones. It is usually the complicated things—making money, forging a career—that lead to prestige and recognition. Yet just how important are prestige and recognition? This is a question rarely asked. Preoccupation with getting ahead is very often done at the expense of our more basic human activities. Perhaps because of this, many people today are going back to basics and seeking out what is primary and basic in human life. Those who do not may be left unsatisfied in life. Without realizing it, they are damaging themselves and often those around them as well. Ask yourself if the means you are using are the most reasonable ones for achieving your ends. The answer is all too often that they are not.

One way of improving an unsatisfying existence is to design a simpler lifestyle. Spend less time on career-oriented activities that serve to increase your material wealth and spend more time on social activities with friends and family, and on physical activity. Cultivate the interests and activities that add to you as a person and increase your enjoyment of life. In the long run, a simple lifestyle leads to a more relaxed and happy existence than a deeply materialistic one.

LIBERATE YOURSELF
FROM THE CAUSE OF STRESS.

If you are to counteract stress, you must free yourself from whatever you find negatively confining. First determine what is keeping you in your "web of stress." Sometimes simply becoming aware of the problem will release you.

If it is another person who is affecting you, you may find it helpful to talk to that person about your feelings. Sometimes this is impossible, and your only course of action may be to put some distance—either physical or psychological—between you and the source of your confinement. Stop thinking about what confines you.

To illustrate the benefits of distance, consider the following example. A twenty-five-year-old married woman, Susan had a strong attachment to her mother without actually realizing it. She *had* to keep house just as her mother had: everything always neat and orderly. However, Susan's husband Jerry did not fit this picture. He was unconcerned with tidiness and was not an especially practical person. Susan's mother criticized Jerry periodically. Then Susan got a job and no longer had the time to keep the house as tidy as her mother expected. This eventually became a source of stress in Susan's life; she felt guilty that the house was not perfect, and rushed home every day to work on it. At the same time, she felt obligated to teach Jerry to live up to her mother's expectations of him. This led to a great many conflicts between husband and wife. He felt pressured, became irritated and depressed, and could no longer concentrate at work.

Susan did not realize that she was attempting to fulfill her mother's demands and expectations, and she could not see that this was the main cause of the stress and tension in her marriage.

However, by establishing a mental and to a certain extent physical distance from her mother over a period of time, she began to improve. Even her relationship with her mother, which had never been particularly good, became better. And from a distance she was finally able to articulate her problem, discuss it with her husband, and overcome it. Life returned to normal.

Such an example is hardly extraordinary. Be alert in your own life to the external pressures that restrict your natural behavior.

LIVE IN THE PRESENT.

People drag the past around with them in the form of guilty feelings, irritations, conflicts, or depression. Others may be so preoccupied with future goals that they simply do not have time to live in the present and solve day-to-day problems; the present disappears in all-consuming thoughts about the past and future. It can be very difficult to free yourself from the constrictions of your past behavior, but try to think only about the positive things in your past and forget about the rest. And remember that life can be viewed as a series of "nows." The future is just a new "now." Try to live only in the present—it's all you have!

By now you should have some idea of the areas in which you are a victim of stress. Many of your specific problems can probably be found, with the appropriate Training Sequences for each, in the next two chapters. You may also have a unique stress-related problem that you wish to solve. Make this problem the central part of your training, following the basic exercises described in Chapter Two. Once you are in a state of deep relaxation, imagine yourself in your stress situation. This will let you begin to associate relaxation, rather than stress, with your problem.

You must also create, in your stress situation, positive thoughts (words, sentences, and images) that help you solve your problem. These positive words, sentences, and images are usually the converse of the negative thoughts you customarily have in this situation. Starting at this point, begin to formulate a Training Sequence.

Let's take a specific example. You are a book editor who is responsible for several books each publishing season, and you find that you have great difficulty meeting your deadlines. The stress and the tension that results from it only make meeting your deadlines even more difficult.

Once you recognize your problem, make a chart in your journal. Write down a description of the problem. List all your negative reactions to the problem and jot down the desired reactions. Finally, formulate an appropriate Training Sequence to help you overcome the problem. For example:

SAMPLE ANALYSIS CHART

PROBLEM SITUATIONS	STRESS REACTIONS	DESIRED REACTIONS
I have too little time to meet my deadlines.	I become nervous.	I am relaxed.
	I become unsure of myself.	I believe in myself.
	I don't believe things will go well.	I know things will go well.
	I become pessimistic.	I look positively at the situation.
	I become irritated.	I am calm and in control.
	I give up easily.	I keep on trying.
	I wander aimlessly and can no longer concentrate.	I take it easy, keep things in proper perspective, and maintain my ability to concentrate. I know I will succeed.

TRAINING SEQUENCE

I am relaxed.
I am confident.
I am optimistic.
I am in control.
I can concentrate.
I can succeed.

Through the simple self-analysis in this chart, you can begin to understand your problem and yourself. You can also begin to take positive, constructive steps to deal with and relieve your stress situations.

4 Reading Your Mind: The Mental Symptoms of Stress

Treating the symptoms of stress before the causes may seem like putting the cart before the horse. Obviously, every symptom has its cause, and the best treatment attacks both at the same time. For most people, however, the symptoms of stress are easier to recognize than the causes, and for this reason we begin the discussion with symptoms. Furthermore, stress symptoms such as nervousness or irritation can actually create stress, becoming a cause of further stress and leading to a series of vicious cycles.

Let's begin. First, remember that your physical training program, whether it is jogging—which is outlined later in the book—or some other exercise mode will greatly alleviate almost all stress symptoms. The following sections briefly describe each symptom of stress, with some suggestions for relieving each. This is followed by the appropriate Training Sequence, to be inserted into your daily training program after the warm-up and basic relaxation exercises. Do not attempt to overcome more than one or two problems at a time at first, and spend at least a week working on the appropriate Training Sequence for each symptom before going on to another. Pick and choose among the sequences and concentrate on those that best suit your own stress situations.

NERVOUSNESS AND ANXIETY.

It is natural to become nervous when facing a new situation: just before making a speech, taking an exam, running a race, or meeting new people.

However, too much nervous tension over a long period can have negative consequences. For example, you may be nervous about an impending business deal, or you may worry about your financial responsibilities. Such nervous tension has a tendency to spread to other areas of your life until you are nervous in nearly all situations without knowing why. This state is called anxiety, the result of many persistent nervous reactions and unresolved conflicts. Eventually, you feel unable to cope with anything.

Regular exercise is one of the best treatments for chronic nervousness, although finding the cause and eliminating it —if there is a specific cause—will clearly cure your nervousness.

TRAINING SEQUENCE

I am breathing deeply and calmly.
My breathing is steady.
My stomach is comfortable and calm.
I feel secure and calm.

IRRITABILITY.

An early symptom of stress is irritability, and especially sensitivity to noise. Loud music or even the sound of the telephone may anger you. This often turns into a vicious cycle. Stress leads to irritability, causing greater stress and eventually causing such physical problems as stomach ulcers or high blood pressure, which make you more irritable. On the other hand, irritability over a short period is common and natural, and should not be taken as a danger signal.

> ## TRAINING SEQUENCE
>
> I am reacting completely calmly.
> I am capable of relaxing completely.
> I understand that irritation doesn't solve anything.
> I am more tolerant.
> I accept the things that are happening around me.
> I am capable of finding constructive solutions.

RESTLESSNESS.

You wander aimlessly about, incapable of remaining calm. You need activity. It is difficult to say just when this otherwise normal reaction becomes a symptom of stress. If it lasts for a long period or happens frequently, be on guard.

Stress-related restlessness usually causes you to work aimlessly, hopping from one thing to another, finishing nothing. At home you cannot sit down and take it easy. Instead, you read the newspaper as fast as possible, preferably while eating. You may start biting your nails, smoking, or developing jittery movements of the hands or feet. Stress makes many people talk too much and too fast.

> ## TRAINING SEQUENCE
>
> I am completely relaxed.
> I have plenty of time.
> My inner tempo is quiet and easy.
> I feel peaceful waves throughout my body.

CHRONIC WEARINESS.

Stress situations often lead to an initial increase in energy, and many people accomplish a great deal when stressed. Yet this also has its negative side. People who have been in high gear for a long time eventually tire easily and exhaust themselves more and more quickly. They burn out. Nervousness associated with stress is especially energy draining; you become increasingly tired at work and may even wake up tired in the morning.

If you have strong psychological defense mechanisms, as described in Chapter 3, you probably also suffer from this kind of chronic weariness, which is not associated with the normal fatigue that follows a hard day's work.

TRAINING SEQUENCE

My body is at rest.
I am completely relaxed.
Everything is comfortable.
My thoughts are clear and calm.
I feel rested.
I am awake and alert.
I feel strong.
I have plenty of energy.

REDUCED PERFORMANCE ABILITY.

Long-lasting negative stress, spontaneous nervousness, and anxiety reduce your mental and physical ability to perform. Driving yourself without rest eventually makes you less capable of working effectively. Acquired negative behavior patterns also prevent you from working to your full potential; you may lack confidence or set only limited goals. Yet you cannot perform well if you are overcome by strong escapist and defense reactions or have a fear of failure. Negative self-esteem, characterized by such thoughts as "I am not smart"; "This will never work"; "Others can do this better than I can"; "I failed the last time I tried"; or "This looks too difficult" will also hinder you.

Chronic weariness and poor concentration are some of the signals of this reduced performance ability. Your psychic energy has been drained away, and your mind, preoccupied with the problems of stress, cannot concentrate at work.

There are several definite things you can do to improve your performance. First, quite simply, try to get enough sleep and stay in good shape. When you are working, make sure that you stay relaxed, even at difficult tasks. Take several short breaks—rest *before* you become tired—and do a few simple relaxation exercises during the day. Make a working plan for yourself and follow it, concentrating on only one thing at a time. When you are not at work make sure you get enough recreation, and do not think about your work when you are resting.

TRAINING SEQUENCE

I can reach my goals.
I dare to set high goals.
I believe in myself.
I accept myself.
I dare to make mistakes.
I keep my sense of humor while working.
I feel relaxed and sure of myself.
I am working confidently.
I am making the most of my resources.
I can concentrate while I work.

ACTION PARALYSIS.

The bad habit of putting things off is quite common. Some typical reactions include such excuses as: "I don't have time"; "I'm not interested"; "I'm not in the mood"; "I'll do it later"; "Things will work themselves out." Eventually you become practically paralyzed, especially when faced with an unpleasant task. The stress triggered by facing the task only makes you more and more paralyzed and you postpone more and more things. You become passive even toward the positive things that might improve your stress situation; you may postpone problem-solving, alleviating boredom, making changes, stopping smoking, cutting down on your alcohol consumption, getting medical check-ups, dieting, or even spending more time with the family.

The passivity can be caused by the fear of failure or change, as well as by energy-draining stress. Change often brings about insecurities.

Many people become action-paralyzed because their standards are too high. Such perfectionists become unable to get anything done, and defend their own paralysis by criticizing others for not being thorough or clever enough, or for being too easygoing, irresponsible, or careless.

This symptom can be treated in some very practical ways: Set up a list of the things you commonly put off doing, and ask yourself why you put these things off. Are other things really more important, or are you afraid of criticism? Also, realize that the problem becomes worse the longer you put it off. It is better to get something done, starting with a very small task, than to get nothing done at all. It might help to create a bit of pressure by telling others what you plan to do.

TRAINING SEQUENCE

I am able to see what my problem is.
I am able to make a decision.
I have decided to take action now.
I can make a choice.
I accept myself and my choices.
I dare to make mistakes.
I am able to tolerate criticism.
I can count on myself.
I won't ignore my problems.
I am confident.
I am action-oriented.
I am secure now; I will make a decision.
I like taking action.

FEAR OF PROBLEMS.

Closely related to postponement is the fear of a problem. Some people react to problems by drawing away from them and worrying that new ones will arise. They develop a "conflict phobia"—an extreme fear of coming into conflict with others—and belittle themselves. They subordinate themselves to others in an unhealthy way.

Problems are a natural part of life. They exist to be solved. They are part of life's challenge. Take a positive and constructive attitude toward your problems instead of worrying about them and avoiding them. In order to solve your problem, you must first analyze it. Define it. Write it down. Set up a self-analysis chart (page 50). What does its solution really involve? What is the worst thing that can happen? How likely is it that this really will happen? Discuss your problem openly with others, and be willing to let them correct you.

Remember, most people tend to exaggerate problems or difficulties. Do not throw the problem out of proportion. Meet it. Be active. Take the initiative.

TRAINING SEQUENCE

I can define the problem.
I have the courage to analyze the problem.
I will find a solution to it.
I have strength and freedom.
I am calm.
I have control over the situation.
I am active and confident.

EXCESSIVE SELF-CENTEREDNESS.

It is natural to be self-centered to some degree. However, stress causes many people to become increasingly involved with themselves and their own problems. Some ponder and brood over their problems to such an extent that they soon become deeply depressed.

Once you have recognized that you are all wrapped up in yourself, you can take some positive steps to break free. Force yourself to become involved with others; listen to what they say. And distract yourself with other things: listen to good music, take up dancing or a sport, go to the movies or theater. In other words, take the initiative.

TRAINING SEQUENCE

I can forget about myself.
I can become involved with others.
I can take the initiative.
I can master any situation.
I am active and free.

LACK OF SPONTANEITY.

When you lose the ability to enjoy life, the world becomes gray. You no longer enjoy the pleasurable things you once did. Stress can create this sorry state, and along with it comes the loss of spontaneity. And when you feel you are not experiencing life to its fullest, you become even more stressed.

To break out of this negative cycle, force yourself to become actively involved with something you enjoy in your spare time, and begin thinking more positively.

TRAINING SEQUENCE

I feel relaxed.
I can take the initiative.
I am active and free.
I am capable of finding positive solutions.
I am spontaneous.
I have things to be happy about.

SOCIAL ISOLATION.

A common stress reaction is listlessness and a desire to be alone. Many people draw away from their friends, becoming apathetic and speaking as little as possible. Actually, such victims of stress are overwhelmed by their own problems, and probably caught in a vicious cycle.

Awareness of this vicious cycle is the first step to breaking out of it. Begin by keeping in touch with your friends and talking to them about your problems. Seek out solutions and activities that you find enjoyable. You might consider joining an organization—a runners' club, health club, discussion group. Take yourself to the movies, theater, a concert, museum, or whatever interests you.

TRAINING SEQUENCE

I dare to take the initiative.
I can find positive things to think about.
I can speak openly with others.
I accept myself.

PHOBIAS.

Long-lasting stress may lead to various phobias. These can be baffling, particularly since they seem unfounded. Most readers will be familiar with and may even suffer from one or another of the clinical phobias, such as claustrophobia, agoraphobia, or hydrophobia (fear of closed spaces, open spaces, and water, respectively). These phobias can sometimes be manifest in unusual and quite specific ways; some people are abnormally fearful of going into stores, riding the subway, or taking an elevator. Others are afraid of heights, of crowded streets, of large dogs, of heavy traffic, or of public speaking. The list is practically endless.

Although many phobias result from stress or unresolved conflicts, this is not always the case. The blame may rest with a specific negative experience; a bumpy plane trip, for example, may cause a fear of flying.

Whatever the cause, phobias are often difficult to overcome, and finding the source of stress- or conflict-related phobias may require the help of a professional therapist. However, you can still work on the symptoms of these phobias to control the anxiety they create. And if the phobia was caused by a negative experience, controlling the symptoms may turn out to be a key to the solution.

Your aim is to feel safe and secure in the situations that bring about anxiety. For two months, train with the basic program. After this, begin to imagine yourself in the situation that creates anxiety (in an airplane, in the water, in a store) while concentrating on remaining relaxed. As soon as you feel tension developing, mentally remove yourself from the situation and concentrate only on becoming calm, relaxed, and secure. When you become completely calm, go back once again to the anxiety-causing situation.

Work on only one situation at a time, beginning with the one that causes you the least amount of anxiety. Again, remember that physical activity tends to inhibit an anxiety reaction. Devise your own Training Sequences, based on the specifics of your phobia, following the guidelines for self-analysis on page 50 and including phrases from basic Training Sequence #4 (page 14).

The mental symptoms of stress can be quite disturbing and difficult to relieve; however, the body's response to stress can be equally debilitating, and no program would be complete without a discussion of the physical symptoms and guidelines for treating them. In the next chapter, we will cover this ground and give you appropriate Training Sequences and exercises to help relieve specific stress-induced ailments.

5 The Body's Message: The Physical Symptoms of Stress

"Listen to your body." Every beginning runner is told this. The body will tell you what you are doing right and wrong. Its performance will reflect your treatment of it. With the proper diet, good sleeping and other habits, and the right amount of exercise, all will be well. But with improper diet, bad habits such as smoking or drinking too much, excessive stress, overuse, or exercising or working too hard, your body will soon break down.

There are several common signals of stress that your body communicates, and once you recognize them, they can be controlled with the mental training program, among other things. However, some of these stress-related signals can have serious consequences, and we will therefore begin our discussion with them.

HEART PROBLEMS.

Stress can cause various types of chest pain and heart disturbance, including pressure or pain in the region of the heart, heart palpitations, and an irregular heartbeat. Stress-related heart pains are typically localized in the left side of the chest, in the area around or a little below the nipple. There may be a stabbing sharp pain that lasts only a few seconds or a duller aching feeling that lasts for several minutes or even longer. There can also be a combination of symptoms. Many people naturally become alarmed when they experience such symptoms, and believe they have developed some form of heart disease. However, this is very often not the case, and the symptoms will disappear when the stress disappears or during physical activity, when the heart must work considerably harder. On the other hand, such symptoms can indicate a serious condition. Should they occur frequently, you should certainly consult your physician.

Heart attacks account for approximately 30 percent of deaths among men and 20 percent among women and an unhealthy lifestyle appears to dramatically increase the risk of heart disease. This lifestyle is characterized by stress, by a constant battle against the clock and striving toward unrealistically high goals, by a poor diet and sedentary habits, and by such other risk factors as smoking, drinking too much. Recent research has shown that regular exercise gives increased protection against heart disease, and especially against hardening of the arteries, therefore decreasing the risk of angina pectoris (see below) or a heart attack. And as we have emphasized earlier, physical activity reduces the level of stress, a definite benefit for the heart. Obviously, too, patients in good physical shape recover from a heart attack more easily and with fewer complications than those in poor shape prior to the attack.

But what is heart disease and how do we recognize its symptoms? Coronary heart disease is caused by atherosclerosis, a condition commonly known as hardening of the arteries (from the Greek *athere*, meaning porridge, and *skleros*, meaning hard). The disease causes a gradual reduction of the blood flow to the heart muscle as well as to other parts of the body, with the result that the supply of oxygen and nutrition may be insufficient for the body's needs, especially during heavy work or exercise. Lack of oxygen in the heart muscle will cause the pain known as *angina pectoris* (Latin *angere*, meaning to strangle, and *pectus*, meaning chest). If an artery closes completely, such as when a blood clot blocks an already narrow artery, a heart attack can occur. The attack actually involves the local death of cells due to a lack of blood supply. This leaves a scar in the tissue.

Although atherosclerosis is normally a long and, to a certain degree, natural process of aging, increasing numbers of younger people are today developing arteriosclerosis.

Typically, persons suffering from angina pectoris feel a constricting, driving pain behind the breastbone, as though a heavy weight were being pressed against the chest. The pain often radiates out to the left shoulder and down the arm into the joints of the hands and fingers. Pain is sometimes also felt in the back, and although it can occur in both sides of the body, is most common on the left side. The pain occurs more frequently after meals and in cold weather.

Angina pectoris is often provoked by physical exertion, such as shovelling snow, heavy lifting, walking or running uphill, or climbing stairs. Sexual activity can also bring on the pain of angina pectoris, and in sedentary people, emotional excitement—irritation, fear, and anger—are the most common provocations. Even watching television may cause such pain to develop.

A heart attack need not necessarily follow from a previous condition of angina pectoris. In many people it occurs completely without warning. The attack itself is experienced as very sudden and strong pain in the middle of the chest. Moreover, while the pain of angina pectoris seldom lasts more than fifteen minutes at a time, the pain of a heart attack often lasts several hours. During this time, nausea, paleness, and cold sweating often occur, accompanied by a general feeling of weakness.

If you are a victim of heart disease or have experienced a heart attack, you can still to a large extent regain your strength and health by systematic training. Physical training will also help to reduce post-heart-attack anxieties and worries about having new attacks. Any exercise program, however, *must* be done under the close supervision of your doctor. Be certain to advise your doctor that you plan to combine mental training with your physical training.

An Ounce of Prevention

If you know you have a healthy heart, there are several things you can do to decrease the risk of heart and artery disease. Start and maintain a regular exercise program; this should take the form of endurance activities such as jogging. Make sure you have a well-balanced diet

·with a relatively low fat content. Do not eat and drink too much. Stop smoking. Reduce the stress in your life. If such things as deadlines, irritations, and overtime work are keeping your life at a high stress level, it would be worthwhile to change this lifestyle and become active in the regular relaxation program described in this book.

HIGH BLOOD PRESSURE.

High blood pressure (also called *hypertension*), an important risk factor in the development of various illnesses—especially heart disease—occurs in about 10 percent of the adult population in the western world. By the age of sixty, this figure increases to 20 percent. Yet it is quite difficult to define absolutely the medical causes of high blood pressure. Relatively few lay people even understand what "high blood pressure" means.

In order for blood to circulate through the body, bringing nutrition to all the body's cells, it must be pushed through the veins and arteries by a certain amount of pressure, produced by the pumping activity of the heart. When the heart muscles contract, blood is pumped out of the chambers into the main artery (the aorta). The pressure under which the blood is pumped from the heart is called *systolic* pressure. When the heart muscles relax, blood that has returned to the heart flows into the chambers. The decreased pressure at which this occurs is called the diastolic pressure. Blood pressure measurements give the relationship of the systolic and diastolic pressures. The measurement is usually taken with the subject in a relaxed sitting or lying-down position. Young, healthy people generally have a systolic pressure of between 115 and 130 mmHg (millimeters of mercury) and a diastolic pressure of about 75 to 85 mmHg, expressed as 115 over 75 (115/75) or 130 over 85 (130/85).

It is difficult to say just where the boundary between normal and high blood pressure lies. Age is one factor that contributes to an increased blood pressure: a blood pressure of 150/95 in a twenty-year-old would call for a closer examination, whereas the same blood pressure in a sixty-year-old would not be considered particularly high. Light to moderate hypertension usually means a blood pressure of from 140/90 to about 160/110.

In about 5 percent of hypertension cases, the high blood pressure is clearly related to diseases of the kidneys, the hormone-producing glands, or the main arteries, among other factors. Heredity and lifestyle also play a role. As with heart disease, specialists agree that smoking, obesity, physical inactivity, poor eating habits, and stress have a definite role in increasing the blood pressure.

The vast majority of persons with light to moderate hypertension will benefit greatly from regular exercise. As with those who have heart disease, the same precautions should be taken, and a doctor's consultation is a must. As a general rule, the intensity of exercise should be moderate, and the activities should be aerobic, such as brisk walking, jogging, running, skiing, swimming, or bicycling. Persons with high blood pressure should avoid such activities as wrestling and weight-lifting, since they can easily bring about a rapid increase in blood pressure. Any training program should progress at a slow pace, and should always include warm-up exercises. The training should never be so hard that it causes pounding in the head or ringing in the ears. Long, relaxed training sessions three times a week are much better than short, intense daily sessions.

If you have seriously high blood pressure, your doctor will probably recommend that you begin a training program only after your blood pressure level is brought under control through medication.

Stress and High Blood Pressure

An immediate reaction to a stress impulse is that the blood pressure rises. Continual stress can eventually lead to chronic high blood pressure. For example, it has been shown that air traffic controllers, who, being responsible for the lives and safety of others, are unquestionably stressed, develop high blood pressure four times more frequently than the average population.

If hypertension is the result of long-lasting stress, regular exercise as well as mental relaxation training can help. Exercising two or three times a week over a six-month period has shown to lead to a decrease of 14 to 16 mmHg in the systolic pressure and of 10 to 12 mmHg in the diastolic pressure. However, if the reduced blood pressure is to remain that way, exercise must continue on a regular basis. Mental relaxation exercises also reduce blood pressure, but to be effective must become a regular part of your daily routine.

TRAINING SEQUENCE

I am completely relaxed.
My heart is beating slowly and calmly.
The blood is flowing calmly around my body.
My heart is working rhythmically and calmly.
My muscles are completely relaxed.

At some time, most people will have experienced less severe symptoms of stress than heart disease or chronic hypertension. These can usually be dealt with quite simply and directly with physical and mental relaxation exercises.

MUSCULAR TENSION.

Stress frequently causes muscle tension. The severity of this depends on both the degree of stress and on how long the stress situation has lasted. Some people can actually feel their muscles tensing, while others feel only the pain resulting from strained muscles. Many people tense their jaw muscles, clamping their teeth together; others tense their legs, neck, shoulders, or back. Stress-induced muscle tension is especially bad when combined with static muscle work—work that requires the muscles to remain in the same position over a period of time, such as typing, various forms of factory work, or hairdressing. Regular and all-round exercises that activate the particular groups of muscles you are having problems with will alleviate muscle tension. The exercises shown here are easy to do at work or at home and are very effective. A specially designed rope ("rolling rope") or a common jumprope with wooden or plastic handles can be used. Regulate the length of the rope by doubling or redoubling around handles. After exercising, stretch the affected muscles for best results.

If your work involves a lot of static muscle work, try to vary your

A tensed arm with fist balled.

A relaxed arm.

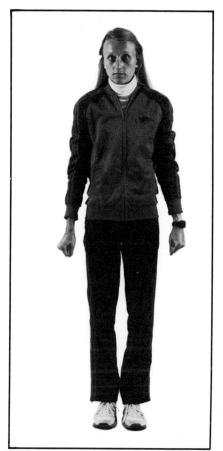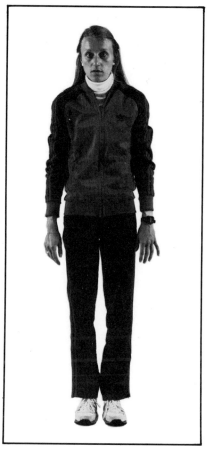

working position and concentrate on keeping the muscles relaxed. Take breaks and stretch and activate the tensed muscles. You should do this even if your muscle tension in unrelated to your work. A simple routine is as follows: Shut your eyes; contract the tensed muscle for approximately three seconds; feel the tension; relax and concentrate on relaxing the muscle as completely as possible for approximately thirty seconds. Alternate in this way between tensing and relaxing for five to ten minutes, preferably several times throughout the day. Carefully notice the difference between the tension and relaxation in the muscles. The point is to become aware of your muscle tensing so that you can later relax the tension on a muscle whenever you wish.

> TRAINING SEQUENCE
>
> The tension in the muscle is disappearing.
> The muscle is completely relaxed.
> The muscle is resting.

HEADACHES.

A normal consequence of long-lasting muscular tension is tension headache. This is commonly related to muscle tension in the neck and head region. (Head and shoulder rolls are effective exercises for this problem; see page 8.) But if the headache varies with the situation, it is most likely caused by psychological stress. Headaches can appear to become worse during the initial phase of your training. If you continue with the training, they normally will be reduced or disappear.

> TRAINING SEQUENCE
>
> I am completely calm and relaxed.
> I am relaxing completely.
> My neck is warm and comfortable.
> My forehead is light and clear.
> The pain in my head is disappearing.

COLD EXTREMITIES.

Muscle tension can reduce the blood flow to muscle cells. In addition, the small blood vessels may decrease in diameter (constrict) as a consequence of the abnormal and chronically increased activation of the nervous system that occurs with constant muscle tension. This impedes the circulation, and the hands and feet feel cold. Activation of the sweat glands, which are abundantly distributed on the palms, on

Hold the rope taut behind your neck.

Pull one arm out to the side as you pull the other behind your neck. Stretch the extended arm back and down.

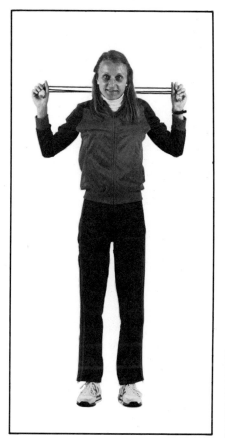
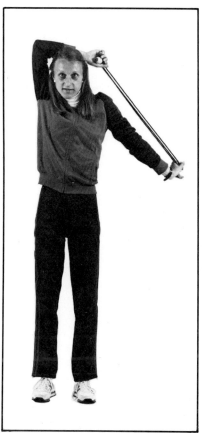

the forehead, and in several other locations may also contribute to this feeling of being cold as the sweat evaporates.

During aerobic activity, the blood vessels in the exercised muscles will automatically widen in response to the body's increased metabolism, and your hands and feet will very soon be warm again. It is even possible that regular aerobic exercise, over a period of time, will reduce the tendency toward stress-induced cold hands and feet.

While doing the mental training exercises, you will probably find that coldness in the hands and feet disappears with systematic relaxation. Use the Training Sequence below, beginning with your hands. In addition, practice the warm-up exercises that are a part of the basic program.

Repeat on the opposite side. Breathe easily and repeat the movement five times, increasing at your own pace.

Stand with your arms behind your back, with a distance of between four and eight inches between the rope handles. Twist your palms outward.

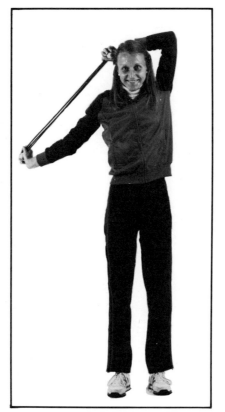
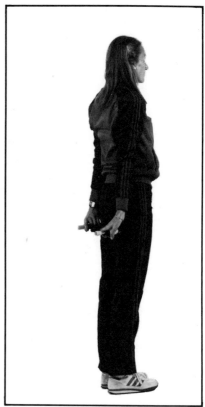

TRAINING SEQUENCE

My hands/feet are warm.
My hands/feet are growing warm.
Warmth is flowing through my hands/feet.
My hands/feet are growing warmer and warmer.

SHALLOW BREATHING.

A common stress reaction is to draw your breathing up into your

Draw your arms up until they are extended straight out from your body.

Bend forward while looking straight ahead, and allow your arms to stretch up over your neck. Return to the original position by reversing all steps. Breathe easily as you do five repetitions. Increase at your own pace.

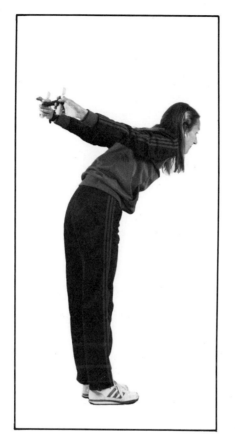
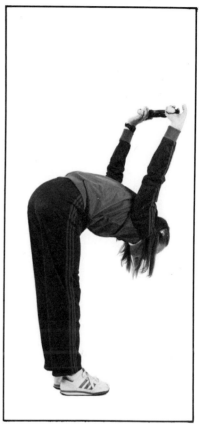

chest. After a while you will probably compensate for this by taking deep breaths or sighing. Normal breathing is both longer and deeper, filling the lungs. Stress breathing may become automatic, making normal breathing increasingly difficult and eventually becoming a major problem.

In your regular exercise program, include a phase of more strenuous activity to give your breathing a real workout: include a few steep hills if you jog, walk, or bicycle; step up the pace if you dance or swim. Do not concentrate on your breathing, but let it work naturally as the intensity of the workout varies. Alternate long and easy with short, hard phases of your workout.

In your mental training program, become aware of your own

Stand with the rope taut behind your neck and your arms at a 45-degree angle.

Stretch your left arm back and down.

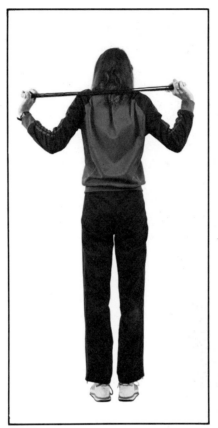
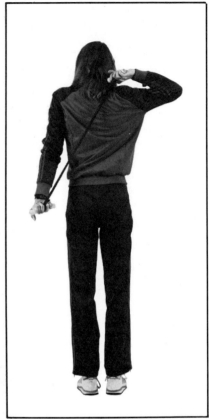

breathing, and recognize the difference between shallow stress-breathing and relaxed breathing. And during the day take time for short breaks (from two to five minutes) during which you concentrate on breathing and practice the following Training Sequence.

TRAINING SEQUENCE

I am breathing deeply and calmly.
My stomach grows as I breathe in.
My lungs are becoming filled with air.

Stretch your right arm back and down.

Immediately lift your left arm up.

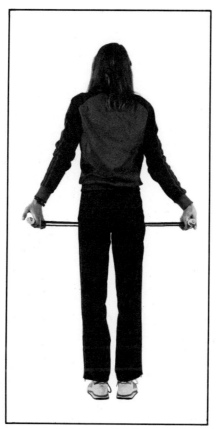 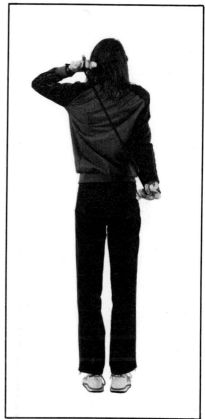

DIZZINESS AND NAUSEA.

Extreme stress and physical tension over a long time can cause nausea, dizziness, or both. You may even throw up or sway or feel that the room is rotating. Such stress reactions can come quite unexpectedly, and frequently occur while you are "relaxing" after a long period of stress.

Following the general mental relaxation program regularly and over a period of time will prevent these annoying symptoms. If, for example, you become dizzy or nauseated under specific circumstances, such as on the street or in an elevator, you can tailor the training program and train yourself directly for that situation (see page 50).

Finally, lift your right arm, returning to the starting position. Work in one fluid motion without stopping at each point. Do five circuits, breathing easily. Increase the number of circuits at your own pace.

Place your right arm behind your back and stretch your left arm over your head.

Pull the rope taut. Pull down with your right arm until it is straight and your left arm is pulled behind your neck. Reverse arms and repeat. Alternate sides, doing the exercise five times on each side. Increase at your own pace and regulate the rope length according to your capabilities.

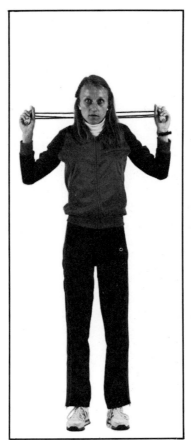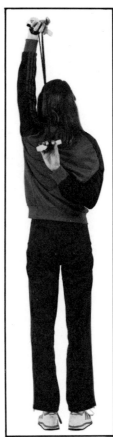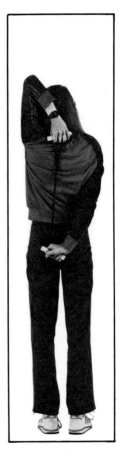

DIGESTIVE DISORDERS.

Stress affects the functioning of the stomach and intestines and can cause painful problems with digestion and bowel movement. For one thing, it brings on the excess secretion of several hormones. In some people this induces a series of internal changes that can eventually develop into ulcers of the stomach and intestinal tract. Unpleasant, negative comments or experiences, irritation, and anger can all lead to contraction of the stomach, the excretion of an abnormal amount of acid, and eventual inflammation of the stomach lining. As many as 10-12 percent of adults in western countries have stomach ulcers, and it is believed that stress is the main cause of two-thirds of these.

A well-balanced diet, rich in fiber, is an important factor in dealing with digestive problems. Although it has not been scientifically proven that regular exercise has a positive effect on intestinal functioning, experience tells us that it does; however, if you already suffer from stomach ulcers, you should consult your doctor before you begin exercising.

In your mental training program, work to determine the cause of an stress-related digestive problem and work systematically on mental relaxation. Besides training with the basic relaxation exercises in Chapter Two, use the following Training Sequence.

TRAINING SEQUENCE

My stomach is completely calm and relaxed.
My stomach is warm.
Warmth is flowing through my stomach.
My stomach is working calmly and comfortably.
My stomach is secure and calm.

SLEEPLESSNESS.

Sleep is the most important energy-building factor known. Good and adequate sleep is an absolute must if we are to function normally. Yet it is difficult to sleep with stressful thoughts and worries running through your head. And too little sleep lowers your resistance to new stress impulses, which only contribute to your problems. The pattern becomes established, a habit is formed, and it is difficult to break.

To deal with insomnia, *do not* become preoccupied with the problem that is causing it, or you will only add to your stress and irritation. Instead, accept the problem and relax. Take a walk or run for an hour or so before you plan on going to bed. Ignore the clock and do not go to bed before you are tired. Once in bed, read something boring without thinking about sleep. The chances are good that you'll soon be asleep.

TRAINING SEQUENCE #1
(before going to sleep)

Sleep doesn't matter at all—it is rest that is important.
I am completely passive.
My thoughts are completely passive.
My eyelids are heavy.
My whole body is heavy and tired.
My eyes are tired and heavy.
I am secure, calm, and passive.
I will sleep deeply and calmly.
I will sleep deeply and calmly throughout the night.

TRAINING SEQUENCE #2
(if you wake up during the night)

I will sleep deeply and calmly the whole night through.
I will sleep deeply and calmly until six o'clock (or whenever
you wish).

MENSTRUAL DIFFICULTIES.

Several studies show that normal menstruation can easily be affected
by stress; it may become irregular or stop altogether for short or long
periods. Reduced fertility can also be a consequence of stress.

A fairly common difficulty is premenstrual syndrome (PMS). PMS
has only recently become the subject of serious study. It is *not* the
result of stress, but in many women can act as a catalyst of stress. One
woman described her premenstrual psychological condition as characterized by such feelings as "Life is nothing by a long uphill climb. I
feel unhappy and miserable. I cry over the slightest thing, and am on
guard about everything. I often go into deep despair after really bawl-
ing someone out." In addition to this, she complained of sore and

Hold the rope with your arms in front of your body.

Stretch your arms up over your head.

Twist your arms behind your back, twisting first to the right . . .

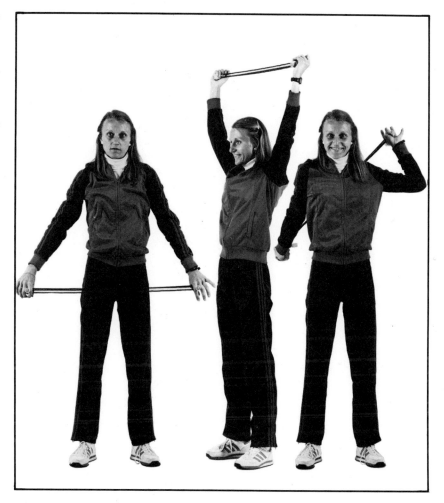

swollen breasts, a weight increase, a generally bloated feeling in the body, and very strong menstrual cramps. This woman is not alone in her complaints.

PMS has been blamed in cases of child abuse and other criminal offenses, and in accidents and suicide. Many tragedies, broken relationships, and unnecessary stress could no doubt have been avoided if those suffering from PMS had been aware of their situation and understood the cause of their trouble.

The most common mental symptoms of PMS are tenseness, irrita-

. . . then to the left.

Pull both arms down behind your back.

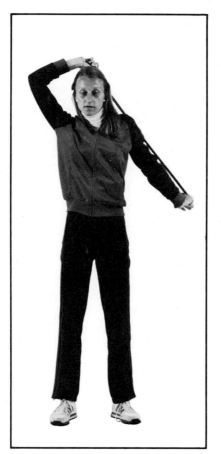
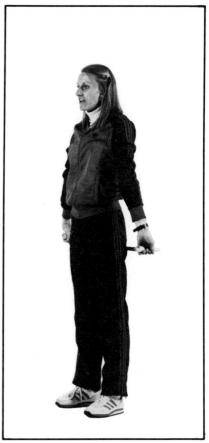

bility, and depression, along with a lack of energy and initiative. The physical symptoms include an increase in weight (as a result of water retention), sore and swollen breasts, headaches, and, at times, severe pains. There is no single accepted explanation for PMS, although its symptoms may occur as a result of reduction of progesterone levels in the blood.

For irregular menstruation and for severe symptoms of PMS, medical treatment can help. Simple awareness of PMS and a basic understanding of the situation will enable you to learn to live with your menstrual cycles. Monitor your body's cycle to find out whether problems seem to be concentrated around a particular number of days

Reverse all the motions and return to holding the rope taut in front of you. Work in a fluid motion and do not stop at each stage. Repeat five times, breathing easily. Increase at your own pace.

Bend forward, keeping your feet a comfortable distance apart.

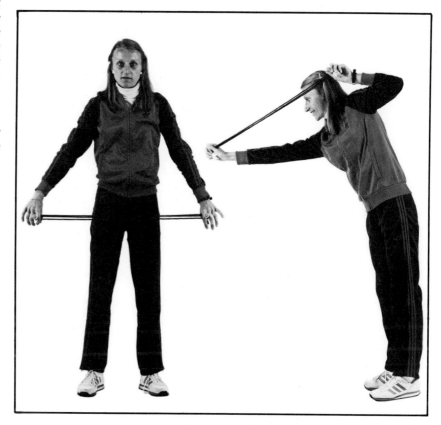

before your period. You can then try to arrange your working schedule and social life accordingly. To reduce the amount of water retention it is also wise to cut down on your salt intake during these days.

Depending on how PMS affects you, devise an appropriate Training Sequence. One of the basic sequences found in Chapter Two may be adequate, or you can adapt one of the more specialized sequences found in later chapters. Because irritability is a common symptom of PMS, it is useful to begin with the Training Sequence on page 37.

SEXUAL IMPOTENCE.

For some people, an especially disturbing consequence of stress is

In a fluid, circular motion, imitate a swimmer's crawl, keeping the rope taut all the while. Repeat five times, then change directions. Breathe easily. Increase at your own pace.

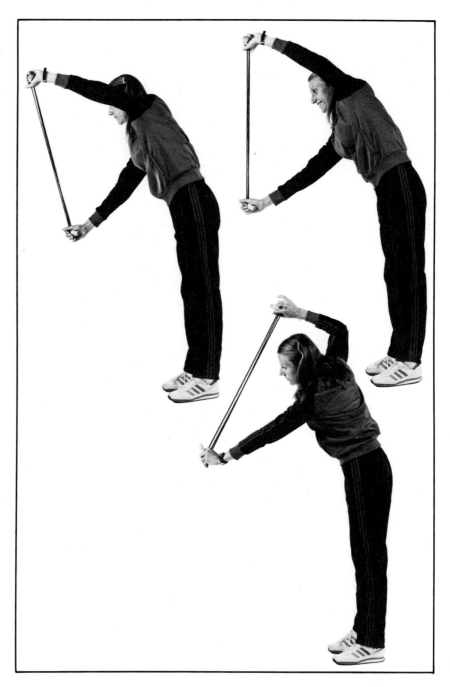

sexual impotence. Anxiety over this condition, and perhaps especially over sexual performance, makes matters even worse. Unconscious mental blocks established during periods of stress and temporary impotence may eventually lead to troublesome long-lasting impotence.

Deep-seated sexual problems may require professional help, but a potency that is reduced by stress usually returns to normal once the stress is eased. Physical activity seems to have a positive effect on potency, since it leads to a greater sense of well-being and a reduced level of stress. An open relationship with your partner, in which you can talk freely about your feelings toward sexuality, is important.

And because mental blocks, anxiety, insecurity, imagined performance demands, and fear of involvement are some of the major causes of sexual difficulties, mental training aimed at reducing anxiety and insecurity can help.

Define your sexual problems and the negative reactions that restrict you—fear, bashfulness, performance anxiety, or mental blocks—and formulate your own Training Sequence with or instead of the one given here.

TRAINING SEQUENCE

I am relaxed and free.
I am active, relaxed, and free.
I dare to give of myself.
I am safe and secure.
I accept myself.

Working on its symptoms, however effective, is still only the beginning of overcoming stress. Nevertheless, it will make you feel better, at least temporarily, and will also give you the freedom you need to analyze your problems and begin to find the probable causes of the stress in your life.

6 Finding the Causes of Stress

Although alleviating the symptoms of stress will make you feel better, the relief may in many cases only be temporary. The symptoms will often return unless you find the cause of the stress and work to control and eliminate it. There is no set formula for determining the cause of stress; the same situation can be stressful to some and not to others. Generally, however, lack of control over the situation is a basic element in causing stress. Also, simply doubting your ability to master a particular situation may be enough to cause stress.

Today there are many situations and relationships that feed insecurities and uncertainties. How you react will determine how stressful a situation will be. By monitoring your reactions, deciding which are negative, and controlling these negative reactions through mental training, you can greatly reduce the stress in your life. In this chapter, rather than examining a list of specific stress situations, we will instead examine the concerns that seem to make situations stressful. In each case, relate the condition to your own situation and, if you can, personalize the Training Sequence according to your own problem (see page 49).

ACHIEVEMENT ANXIETY.

Today's society is strongly achievement oriented. Beginning in school, we are taught to value success, competence, a good social position, material wealth, status, and the opinion of others. Many people come to overemphasize the importance of achievement; they overwork themselves, often developing stress from overstimulation and becoming excessively afraid of making mistakes or seeming foolish.

What, then, is positive achievement? Working toward realistic goals gives meaning to your life. Success or failure depends largely on the goals you have set, the demands you make on yourself, and the importance you put on the expectations of others. If you live up to your own expectations you will feel comfortable with yourself, even if your achievements themselves are not overwhelming. Yet in some cases, even though you do an excellent job at something, you will feel disappointed and stressed if it is not the goal you set for yourself. Many successful people feel they are underachieving. Their goals and expectations become impossibly high.

Other people are actually "afraid" of doing well. They may be afraid of standing out in the crowd or of extra demands being made on them if they do well. They may simply not want to take chances, or may feel they are stealing success from others, thus developing a guilty conscience. Such people trivialize success by saying: "It was just luck. The others did all the work; I just went along for the ride." Another common reaction is to reject compliments. Such a defeatist attitude can cause us to neglect our potential.

People who suffer from achievement anxiety eventually become passive and do not dare to attempt anything at all. Security overrides action.

To break out of the overachievement habit, be constructive in your attitude toward criticism. Seek it out, remembering that no one is always perfect. But remember too that jealousy—rather than constructive judgement—is a frequent motive behind criticism. There are always people who will dislike your successes and enjoy your fiascos. Free yourself from the social ties and people that give you achievement anxiety.

Remember, no one can go through life without making mistakes; learn to accept yours. And take the time to enjoy your achievements and successes. Concentrate on your earlier successes and forget your past blunders; do not allow them to hinder your future successes. In order to reach your goals, you must believe in them, but remember to accept your failures along the way. Tailor a Training Sequence to suit your own expectations or use the one given here.

TRAINING SEQUENCE

I believe in myself.
I dare to do poorly once in a while.
I am brave.
I can free myself from the judgement of others.
I am secure and calm.
I can tolerate criticism.
I seek out criticism.
I am open to criticism.
Everybody makes mistakes.
I am confident and secure.
I dare to take chances.
I accept the uncertain.

ACTIVITY IMBALANCES.

Occasionally everyone experiences a period of high levels of stimulation. Everything becomes chaotic, too many things are happening, there is too much noise, too much fuss, too many telephone calls, too many people, too many deadlines, too much pressure for time, and too many appointments and meetings. Such excessive stimulation causes stress overload. The best cure in such cases is solitude, rest, and relaxation. This simple solution, however, can be difficult. A steady stream of thought works on in our minds, impeding rest and even sleep. Restlessness only makes it more difficult to wind down. Long-lasting stimulation can eventually become almost a necessity; like a drug addict, you feel the need for constant stimulation. Eventually, you begin to work ineffectively, jumping from one thing to the next without finishing anything. Typically, people who suffer from overstimulation stress cannot handle leisure situations well. Weekends and vacations are ordeals.

Yet people thrive on variety, and monotony and understimulation can be just as stressful as overstimulation. You may feel that you are not taking advantage of your talents; your work may be monotonous and repetitious, challenging only a small part of your potential, and you may have little say in how the work is to be done. The job becomes stressful and meaningless, and the chances of your dropping out of the workforce are high. Nervous disorders, insomnia, and the use of medication are greater among people whose work is boring than among those with interesting work. Other candidates for understimulation stress are housewives and recently retired or otherwise unemployed people.

The treatments for both over- and understimulation are based on constructive activity and relaxation.

Those in the throes of overstimulation should begin by making a working plan and following it. Set priorities: the most important and the least pleasant tasks should be done first. While you work, concentrate only on the present, the task you are doing now. Put away everything else that will remind you of the work you have not yet done. It is not usually catastrophic if you do not manage to do everything you should have done. Try to imagine the worst thing that can happen if you do not finish your task; are the consequences so serious that you are willing to sacrifice your health to avoid them? Also, the more upset, worried, and irritated you get, the less work capacity you will have, so do not forget to keep your sense of humor even when you have much to do. While working, use the relaxation and resting techniques that you have been learning. Make sure to relax in your free time: listen to music, go to the movies or theater, or otherwise distract your mind from its problems and engage it with other things.

TRAINING SEQUENCE FOR
OVERSTIMULATION

I have a calm inner tempo.
I work with ease and concentration.
I work at one task at a time.
I can forget the past and the future.

I work in the present.
I have command of my situation.
I work with a good conscience.
I accept myself.
I work with a sense of humor.
I accept that not everything can be done perfectly.
I work without irritation and aggression.
I am calm.
I can accept criticism.

People who are understimulated may be able to break the tedium even if their jobs are monotonous. They must first recognize whether the problem exists because they are afraid of change. Many people keep the same dull job, eat the same foods, dress the same way, and follow unvarying daily routines simply because they are afraid of taking a chance on something new. They approach new experiences with a negative attitude. Yet their own boredom, which also bores others, causes them enormous stress.

If you think this may be you, check it out by answering the following questions: How long has it been since you had an emotional experience that you found pleasant or surprising? Do you always choose to do exactly the same things every day? Is this necessary? Does it make you feel more secure? Do you explore new feelings or do you cling to the intellectual/emotional feelings you are most comfortable with? Do you always need a very good reason for doing something unusual? Your answers will tell you whether it is time for action. Force yourself to seek out new surroundings, new activities, and new people. Do something spontaneous. Try out new ideas at work. Surprise your spouse! Because your own negative attitude determines whether or not you will be bored, try to be open-minded, to make the best of any situation. By using your imagination and intelligence, you may be able to turn something that you find boring—even your job—into something interesting.

TRAINING SEQUENCE FOR
UNDERSTIMULATION

I am using my imagination.
I am discovering what it is I really feel like doing.
I make the most of my situation.
I can solve my problem of boredom.
I take the initiative.
I understand my situation and am doing something about it.
I dare to be active.
I can break the tedium.
I enjoy discovering new things.
I am taking advantage of my capabilities.
I dare to seek out stimulating surroundings.

SELF-INFLICTED PRESSURE.

Many people make unreasonable demands on themselves, not distinguishing between what is important and what is trivial. The world becomes a web of duties and obligations, and when they fail to meet their responsibilities they wind up feeling guilty and adding even more stress to their lives.

If you fall into this category, it is likely that your conversation—even your inner conversation—is liberally sprinkled with "must" and "should." You probably have very rigid ideas about the order in your life and in the lives of those around you, and follow either your own learned habitual patterns or society's conventions: women must not ask men out; housework can be done only by women; gardening is done by men. You are concerned with what is "right" and what is "wrong": the right clothes, the right schools, the right food, the right opinions, the right friends.

You may feel that only you can do a certain task properly, or make the right remark. Eventually, you will be unable to live up to these too-high expectations. Soon you are punishing yourself for not accomplishing the things you think are important. In the long run, self-punishment can become systematic; you can no longer see the difference between what is important and what is not, or reflect on your situation objectively and philosophically. You probably, and wrongly, feel that other people expect you to fulfill your own unrealistic expectations.

Treat this condition somewhat like the achievement anxiety described earlier. Make a list of your obligations, now matter how large or small they may be. Decide which ones are important to you and which are really quite trivial. Are *any* of them important enough to make you sacrifice your health and well-being? Which create more problems than they solve? Make an effort to eliminate these, along with the ones that are not really all that important. Decide which of your obligations create conflicts and irritations you inflict on others. Try to control these. Next, how many of your obligations are the result of other people's expectations? Discard them—they do not belong to you anyway.

TRAINING SEQUENCE

I see my own situation.
I see my obligations.
I see which ones bother me.
I can free myself.
I have a good conscience.
I accept myself without my unreal obligations.
I feel free.
I make my own decisions.

UNCERTAINTY.

Insecurity may well be the most frequent cause of stress. And contributing to the feeling of insecurity is the lack of stability and permanence in modern life; society's constant flux means a steady stream of new and unfamiliar situations and conditions. Uncertainty about the immediate future—about your economic state, standard of living, threatening world crises—and about your ability to master a particular situation will almost always cause stress. Thus, even though many people are amazingly resilient and adapt to new environments and circumstances, there are limits to the amount and frequency of change and uncertainty they can tolerate before experiencing negative stress.

Your attitude toward change will largely determine the intensity of the stress reaction you experience. Some people welcome and seek out varied stimulation while others tend to shun change. The seekers often try almost any new activity, taking risks, looking for challenges and excitement, and experimenting with themselves and their surroundings. The shunners are just the opposite, needing stability, quiet, and few challenges. In general, the seekers lead healthier, more positive and stress-free lives than the shunners. Being oriented toward looking for change and meeting new challenges, seekers face the future without anxiety and concern. They also have a strong feeling of control over any situation they find themselves in. They see problems as challenges that need solutions, and not as potential disasters.

It is possible to learn a seeker attitude by practicing your mental training. Define and list the situations that make you feel insecure. Ask yourself again: What is the worst thing that can happen? How likely is it that this will really happen? Learn to accept the unavoidable so that it does not become a constant source of stress. Use your energy on things you can change, not on the unchangeable. Remember that it is natural to feel insecure, that everyone appears more secure than they really are. Recognize and accept your insecurities. By doing this you will help to reduce them. And do not let your insecurity itself become a source of insecurity.

The unknown is a challenge to be met with a positive attitude. Concentrate on the positive aspects of a situation rather than the negative. Take the initiative to overcome the unknown.

TRAINING SEQUENCE

I feel safe.
I feel secure.

I dare to meet new challenges.
I meet challenges with calmness and strength.
I can find constructive solutions.
I can find constructive alternatives.
I can tolerate the unknown.
I like the unknown.
I am confident.

WORRYING.

Negative thoughts create negative feelings, and worrying causes stress in many people. There seems to be no limit to the sources of worry: jobs, the future, the weather, bills, aging, appearance, behavior, and other people's opinions are just a few. Some people consider worrying to be a sign of responsibility. They feel more mature when they are plagued by their concerns. It becomes a habit, a bad one.

Only constructive action—not worry—can solve your problems. Worry can cause action paralysis. To break out of a bad pattern of worrying, begin by listing all the things—however trivial—you worry over. Strike out those things you absolutely cannot change, such as weather, and the behavior of others, and strike out the trivialities. Life is too short to waste on such things. Try to put yourself and your problems in proper perspective. Tackle only one problem at a time. And while you do, enjoy what you have instead of worrying about what you do not have, what you have accomplished rather than what you have not. Look forward to the opportunities awaiting you in the future instead of dwelling on the negative things that might happen. Keep your mind and body active, and practice your mental training regularly.

TRAINING SEQUENCE

I dare to live now.
I have a positive attitude toward my problems.
I am free of worries.

GUILT.

When you choose something that your conscience tells you is wrong, you inevitably experience a feeling of guilt. Your conscience is largely based on what others have taught you about right and wrong, about how you should or should not behave. Parents, teachers, and peers all influence the shaping of conscience. Many people also devise their own set of rules and standards, which they then feel guilty for breaking. Such things as spending time on themselves, allowing others to lend a hand, and even feeling any kind of pleasure may produce guilt, which supersedes any positive effects these circumstances may have brought. Even trivial things in everyday life plague the conscience: not finishing a task on time, not having dinner ready on time, not keeping the house spotless.

Guilt, however, will only make you preoccupied with your past mistakes and incapable of functioning in the present. It can also be a way of attracting attention and sympathy. And inflicting guilt is a handy way of controlling one's children, spouse, or colleagues. Recognize any efforts of others to control you in this way.

Decide what causes a feeling of guilt in you and whether the cause is well founded. Very often it is unjustified, coming from a too-rigid set of values. Similarly, wrong values may be making you feel too much guilt. Remember, feeling guilty about mistakes is destructive; *learning* from them is constructive and positive. Recognize the difference.

If you decide that your guilty conscience is well founded, formulate a plan to change your behavior and improve the situation. Solving the problem that causes your guilt is far better than learning to live with a guilty conscience. Remember that you cannot change the past but that you *can* do something about the present. So live in the present, do not think about the past or future. Find what is positive about today, and do not try to solve all of your problems in one day.

TRAINING SEQUENCE

I can find the cause of my guilty conscience.
Guilt doesn't help me.

I can solve my problems.
I dare to take up my problems.
I am calm and relaxed.
I am free and open.
I dare to talk about my conscience.
I can free myself from my guilty conscience.
I can keep my guilty conscience at a distance.
I can solve future problems rather than feel guilty about them.
I learn from my mistakes and act accordingly.

ROLE PLAYING.

It is natural to play various roles in your life. You may be a parent, spouse, consumer, and boss in the course of a single day. Different situations require different responses. As a neighbor you behave in one way, as a worker in another way, and as a lover in still another. Think about your behavior in your various roles. Are you different?

Since the pressure to fulfill various roles is so strong, your roles have quite a firm psychological hold on you. Some can function as negative stress factors in your life: the superwoman role, the conformist role, the dominant man role, the dependent woman role, the successful man role, and so on. These are usually roles that conform to the expectations others have of you.

Everyone depends on other people to some degree, but overdependence means that your own personality almost disappears. You do *exactly* and *only* what others expect and demand of you. You cannot tolerate others disliking you or disagreeing with you or challenging your opinions. A typical reaction is to stop trusting yourself and to always seek the advice of others first, waiting to speak until hearing their opinions and changing yours to suit theirs.

Especially susceptible to such dependence are people whose parents have been extremely strict, demanding unquestioning obedience and submissiveness. Women at home also seem particularly prone to patterns of negative role-playing. They become totally dependent on the expectations of others; they must fulfill the expectations of their children, husbands, or parents—and often those of all three; they must be entertaining, helpful, and cheerful. Their own schedules and interests are subordinate to those of others.

It takes courage and great mental effort to break out of negative roles, Analyze the roles you play. You will find that some make you feel secure while others cause you stress. List them accordingly. Which ones make you feel stressed? What demands of others do you find unpleasant? What expectations make you feel stressed? When you have done this, you should be aware of the negative roles you play.

Your own behavior may also contribute to others' expectations of you. If it does, it also affects you negatively. Try first to change your own behavior and give others time to get used to the change. Discuss your roles and changes with friends; role-changing requires a change in their attitude too. Avoid people who try to keep you locked in your negative roles. If it is impossible to avoid such people physically, try at least to do so mentally.

Realize that you cannot always agree with everyone, and that not everyone is going to like you. Be prepared to argue for your opinions if necessary, and be assertive in social situations. Almost all issues have arguments for and against. Do not let this stop you from taking a stand.

TRAINING SEQUENCE

I am free and independent.
I trust myself.
I dare to reveal myself.
I stand by my opinions.
I accept others' disagreement.
I accept making mistakes.
I cannot avoid making mistakes now and then.

I am sure of myself.
I feel good about myself.

EMOTIONAL STARVATION.

There is a basic human need for love, affection, and acceptance. Without these necessities, a child's emotions do not develop properly—a defect that is carried far into adulthood. Such emotional starvation is a common affliction in today's society, where divorce and stressed families are common. Without doubt this plays a major role in causing stress.

For many people, a stumbling block to treating this problem is the difficulty they have in recognizing that even they have these needs. As long as you do not accept your emotional needs, you will do nothing to seek fulfillment for them. The inability to accept love and affection may also mean the inability to give it. Some people even have such an aversion to the idea of love that they react negatively to the word itself; they become embarrassed, disgusted, withdrawn, or awkward when the topic of love comes up.

In general, emotional needs are difficult to express to other people. Fear of rejection, for one thing, can prevent you from being open. This means that others must guess your needs, and obviously they can guess wrong. Even those closest to you may therefore disappoint you simply because they misinterpret your unspoken needs.

You must learn to be open. Recognize and accept your emotional needs. And accept the needs of others. Seek out people and surroundings that help to satisfy your needs, that make you feel loved and important. Avoid people and surroundings that leave these needs untouched. Be willing to give love and affection without expecting it in return. Take care of your friends, give them praise and encouragement, and try to make them feel good about themselves and about you. Love is not only to be received—it is also something to be given.

> **TRAINING SEQUENCE**
>
> I accept my need for love.
> I am open.
> I am free.
> I am not afraid to give love.
> I am not afraid to receive love.

Up to this point, we have been dealing with problems—with recognizing and alleviating the negative symptoms and causes of stress. But as you are undoubtedly aware, this is only part of the program. To be truly healthy, you must establish positive diet and exercise regimens and practice them as faithfully as you do the mental training programs.

7 The Keys to Better Health

No matter how conscientious you are about maintaining a mental training program, it will not be truly effective unless combined with physical training and good general health maintenance. Begin by monitoring what you put into your body: what you eat and drink and how much, and the pills and other medications you take. If you still smoke, *now* is the time to take a hard, critical look at a harmful habit.

DIET: YOUR FOOD IS YOUR MEDICINE.

It is widely accepted that diet is the foundation of health and physical well-being, and provides the basis for growth. Yet just what constitutes a reasonable and healthy diet? Myths about food abound; books, newspapers, and magazines constantly tout fad diets and new and exciting advances in the field. Much of the advice given seems contradictory and, in general, questionable.

A sensible diet consists of a balance of seven essential substances: carbohydrates, fat, proteins, minerals, vitamins, water, and fiber.

Carbohydrates and fat are the body's main sources of energy. Protein is used mainly for the development and maintenance of cells and tissues. Minerals and vitamins are essential for the functioning of nerves and muscles, and also interact with the enzymes that speed up important chemical reactions in the body. Additionally, minerals build up and maintain cells and tissues in the bones and teeth, among other structures. The various vitamins are chemically different, each having a specific function to fulfill in the body.

Water is necessary for maintaining the proper concentration of various substances within and around the cells. Fiber, or "roughage," the indigestible particles in the cells of food plants, reaches the end of the intestinal system almost unchanged and aids in the normal digestion process; fiber is found in grain products, vegetables, and fruits.

All of these nutrients can be obtained in adequate quantities by eating food from each of the four main food groups every day.

	FOOD	*NUTRIENTS*
Group I	Bread made with whole-grain wheat; grain products such as cereals, rice, and corn.	Carbohydrates in the form of starch; protein, iron, and other minerals; B vitamins, vitamin E, and fiber.
Group II	Milk and other dairy products such as cheese and yogurt.	Protein; fat; calcium, phosphorus, iron, and other minerals; vitamins A and D, B vitamins.
Group III	Potatoes; all kinds of vegetables including legumes (peas and beans), fruit, and berries.	Carbohydrates; iron and other minerals; vitamins A and C, and fiber.
Group IV	Meat, poultry, fish, and eggs.	Protein; fat; iron and other minerals; B vitamins.

The ideal relationship between the major components of the diet should be carbohydrates, 55 to 60 percent of the total energy consumed; fat, 30 to 35 percent; and protein, 10 to 15 percent. Most people will need to increase their consumption of carbohydrate foods, such as whole-grain breads and other grain products, rice, peas, beans, fruit, and vegetables, while decreasing their dietary intake of fat-rich foods.

Diet Tips

Fat is hidden in many meats and meat products—such as hot dogs, bologna, and pâté—as well as in whole milk, rich salad dressings, sauces, and cakes. Be alert, for the list is long. Even several varieties of fish are high in fat, including herring, mackerel, sardines, bluefish, and salmon. However, fish is a better choice, since all fish contain unsaturated fats and are rich in vitamins A and D. Other fat-rich foods are often poor in vitamins, minerals, and protein.

Milk provides protein and is the most important source of calcium, which is essential for the building of bones and teeth. It also contains many vitamins, including most of the B vitamins. The more regularly you exercise, the more milk you can drink. But be aware that whole milk contains about 32 grams of fat per quart. This may be up to half your daily fat allowance, which means that you have to cut out fats from other sources. A better choice is skimmed milk, with only 4 grams of fat per quart and most of the same nutrients that are found in whole milk. Skim milk does have less vitamin A than whole milk, since, being fat soluble, this vitamin is skimmed away with the fat.

Some people cannot tolerate or do not like milk. For them, cheese is a good alternative. Its nutritional value is the same as that of milk.

Vegetables and fruit should be eaten in as natural a state as possible, since cooking and canning reduces the mineral and water-soluble vitamin content of these foods. Freezing, however, does not lead to any substantial loss of nutrients.

Fiber can be added to your diet simply by eating more whole-grain breads, or in the form of bran, which can be bought in loose form as bran flakes or cereals or in the form of baked goods such as bran breads, crackers, and crisps. An addition of 20 to 30 grams of bran daily is a sensible way to begin your diet.

If you plan on changing your diet, remember that your stomach and intestines will need time to adapt. Changing over too quickly to more natural, less refined food and more coarse-grained products, vegetables, and fruits may cause temporary flatulence and stomach rumbling. Take your time—several weeks if possible—in developing new eating habits.

Women have a greater need for iron than men, and many women should supplement their dietary intake of iron. Iron is found naturally in such foods as liver, kidneys, beef, leafy green vegetables, whole grains, and grain products. The iron in bread and grain products is better absorbed if eaten with foods containing vitamin C.

Dietary Supplements

It is difficult to give an exact definition of "health food." If your diet is deficient, any food that improves it can be considered a health food. Yet the term "health food" has come to be associated with an extensive and confusing array of special products—dietary supplements—that are often described as "necessary" for insuring a healthful diet and life. The information provided with or about these products is often unclear, questionable, or downright false. There is no evidence that such products have any effect at all on people who follow a well-balanced diet.

In recent years, special diet supplements have been tailored for athletes. Many falsely claim to build muscles, increasing the user's performance ability or burning off fat. Do not be fooled. Your diet will surely be healthy if it is based on the four food groups, in well-balanced combination, as recommended in the guidelines already discussed.

SMOKING: AN UNKIND FRIEND.

We cannot talk about the keys to better health without talking about smoking. Millions of people voluntarily fill their lungs with tobacco smoke containing approximately three thousand harmful substances. A single cigarette produces 5 billion particles, each about two-thousandths of a millimeter in size.

The dangers of smoking are becoming better documented and better understood. Early in 1982, the United States Surgeon General termed smoking the number one cause of death in this country. The list of smoking-related problems is long and depressing. On the other hand, the list of advantages gained when you quit smoking is also long, but not at all depressing:

- A restoration of the lungs' defense system against unwanted air particles and harmful substances.

- Less resistance to the passage of air through the lungs.
- A dramatic reduction in the chances of getting various types of cancer.
- A reduced risk of emphysema, chronic bronchitis, and other lung ailments.
- An increased ability of the lungs to deliver oxygen to the blood.
- A reduced risk of heart and artery diseases.
- Enhanced taste sensations and a better appetite.
- A normal reaction to various medications. (It has been shown that a smokers' reactions to medication are often reduced.)
- Better digestion.
- A better sense of smell.
- Fresher breath.
- Increased stamina.
- Better sleep.

However, while it is all well and good to recognize the dangers and to want to stop smoking, taking positive action is difficult. You may even have tried stopping a few times but without success. Needless to say, strong motivation is essential, but will power may not always be enough. Today, there are any number of "smoke-ending" groups to help people conquer the habit. To find out which ones are active in your area, check with your local hospital, chapter of the American Lung Association or American Cancer Society, or your physician.

If you are unwilling or unable to join such a group, you can still follow a program to stop smoking. In order to succeed, your unconscious must learn to take a more negative attitude toward smoking, and the following step-by-step approach should help you in this task.

A Two-Phase Program to Stop Smoking

As with other difficult habits, it is easiest to quit smoking if you do so with a group of like-minded people. If at all possible, follow this program with one or more of your friends, and plan on meeting daily or at least several times a week in the beginning.

Phase One should last for about a month, although you can decide how much time you will need for this educational part of the program. During this time, you should not make any efforts to cut down on smoking. Smoke as you always have—according to the "principle of desire." At your meetings, concentrate on in-depth discussions of the hazards of smoking and its effect on your body. Begin with what you already know, and add to this knowledge by researching the subject. Accumulate and circulate anti-smoking literature among the members of your group. The American Cancer Society and the Heart Association chapter in your area can supply you with literature. A research library is another good source. Learning about the dangers and negative aspects of smoking will help you to develop a negative attitude toward it.

You should also freely discuss your own emotional reaction to the thought of quitting. How important is smoking to you? How dependent are you on it? How does your life revolve around the habit? Tell your family, friends, and colleagues that you are following a five-month program to stop smoking, and remind them of this from time to time, especially during Phase Two. They will be more sympathetic to your moods if they understand the problems you are having.

On your own, during the day, repeat the Training Sequence below and add to or subtract from it according to your own situation. Concentrate on deep breathing techniques (see page 9).

TRAINING SEQUENCE—PHASE ONE

I am relaxed.
I dare to quit smoking.
I am breathing freely.
I am calm.
I can quit smoking.
I am alert.
I am free from the desire to smoke.
The decision is my own.

After a month or so you are ready to begin Phase Two. Now you must start to cut down on the number of cigarettes you smoke. Do not worry—it is going to be a very gradual process. First, depending on how heavy a smoker you are and how gradually you want to change the habit, set a target date for your absolute last cigarette. Next, calculate your weekly comsumption of cigarettes and figure out how many cigarettes you have to eliminate each week in order to reach zero on your target date. Then write down the situations in which you most enjoy or need a cigarette: After dinner? At work? With coffee? At a party? During a meeting? With cocktails? When you are worried or unhappy? Arrange the list in order, from the least to the most difficult situations to get through without smoking.

Begin Phase Two by cutting out cigarettes in the situations at the top of your list, in which you feel least dependent on the smoking habit, and each week add one or more situations, working your way down the list. Do not try to work on too many situations at once, and if necessary, revise your list. Continue to have regular meetings, frequently at first, with your group. Discuss your progress and setbacks, and your reactions—positive as well as negative—to these situations. What activities begin to become more pleasurable without the burden of smoking? In what ways do you feel better? What activities (such as bicycling, walking, or jogging) can you now do and enjoy that you could not really enjoy before you began your non-smoking program? Remember also to discuss your reactions with your family and friends, especially if you are following the program on your own. Expect to feel nervous and irritable at first, and be sure to warn family members and friends when you do. Eventually, you will be more relaxed than you were as a smoker.

Repeat the Phase One Training Sequence as often as possible during the day, especially when you feel the urge for a cigarette. Add to it from the sequence below.

TRAINING SEQUENCE—PHASE TWO

My mind is clear.
My lungs are clear.
I am strong enough to stop smoking.
I am no longer dependent.
I am master of my situation.

> I have will power enough to stop smoking.
> I can fill my lungs with fresh air.

Some people develop weight problems after they quit smoking, and this can become quite discouraging. Many feel that it is a matter of choosing between the lesser of two evils—smoking or gaining weight. The best way to avoid a weight problem is to exercise regularly during your anti-smoking program. Exercise also reduces the uneasiness and restlessness that many people feel as they give up smoking.

DRINKING HABITS.

Alcohol is generally used for relaxation and the relief of anxieties and insecurities. The danger lies in habitual drinking that becomes excessive and often results in a dependence on alcohol. And like smoking, drinking too much too often causes a long, depressing list of health problems. As in many other areas of life, the difference between individual reactions to alcohol is great, and some people seem to tolerate the negative effects of alcohol better than others.

If you drink, it is best to do so only on special occasions, and these do not include moments when you feel depressed or otherwise stressed in some way. Using alcohol as an antidote to stress can easily lead to dependence. Instead, drink only with others—at dinner parties, get-togethers with friends, or cozy Saturday evenings at home.

"A dram is good for the heart," says an old adage in folk medicine, and recent research indicates that there may be some truth to this; small amounts of alcohol may be beneficial. Small amounts of alcohol also break down social and psychological inhibitions and may therefore produce a general feeling of openness and well-being. Many people also experience heightened creativity under the influence of alcohol. Yet it is extremely difficult to find the right balance between the positive and negative effects of alcohol, and the negative effects are all too often the dominant ones.

Mental training is a far better way to cope with stress, depression, and your inhibitions. You can use the basic training sequences found in Chapter 2 and, if necessary, devise your own sequence to solve any minor or developing problems you may have with alcohol. The Training Sequence on page 89, designed to help curb pill use, can easily be adapted to form the basis for an alcohol-targeted Training Sequence. The sequence is not guaranteed to cure a drinking habit, but it can help you to control the habit and perhaps to discover the causes.

TRANQUILIZERS AND STIMULANTS.

Increasing numbers of people are turning to drugs to solve stress-related problems. Pills in particular appear to provide security and an easy answer to day-to-day problems; since 1970, for example, the consumption of tranquilizers has risen dramatically despite the great deal of negative publicity that has been given to them. Of course, in some cases, drugs are necessary aids in the treatment of a psychological problem. Their effect, however, often diminishes in time, and may ultimately disappear—a phenomenon known as tolerance. The level of tolerance to a drug will depend on the drug as well as the individual's reaction to it. In many cases, however, increasingly large doses of a drug are needed in order for it to have any effect.

Both sleeping pills and tranquilizers can have relatively serious side-effects. Many of these drugs are eliminated from the body slowly, often causing dizziness, loss of coordination, poor memory, and slowed reactions. In some people, the continuous use of such drugs may also lead to shaking hands, depression, stomach problems, and constipation. And with the larger doses needed to maintain an effect with prolonged use of these drugs, the more serious the consequences will be.

The abuse of pills demands action, preferably in cooperation with others, in seeking the cause of your problem. To start with, do not carry your problems around with you for so long that you become dependent on drugs. Admit that you have a problem and seek help for it. Neither suppressing it nor making excuses for it is going to solve it.

Mental training can often help you to discover the cause of a drug-related problem and to control the anxiety and nervousness that encourage you to use pills. Only long and systematic training can bring about positive results. You must make mental training part of your daily routine. It can become a positive substitute for the harmful habit of pill consumption,

If you have already developed a dependency, you may need professional help, beginning with a consultation with your doctor, a psychologist, or a psychiatrist. Under his or her direction, you can practice basic training and specialized mental training to help you lose or prevent a dependency on pills.

TRAINING SEQUENCE

I dare to look at my problem.
I will reach my goal.
I am secure and free.
I have control over my problem.
I can be completely free from dependency.
I can liberate myself from pills.
I am secure and happy without pills.
I am more secure and more sure of myself without pills.

With training, the good habits you begin to form will automatically make you feel better physically. And physical well-being will naturally spill over to your mental well-being. Exercising control over your body helps you get into the habit of discipline, of seeing yourself as in control of your life. However, health maintenance not only involves monitoring what you put into your body, but also how you use your body. The next chapter gives you another essential key to good health, tells you how to test your fitness level, and outlines a three-phase exercise program for beginners.

8 Life Is Movement: Training for Your Health

The belief that regular physical activity prevents disease and degeneration, improves health, and lengthens life is as old as mankind itself. As early as the fourth century B.C., Hippocrates said that what is used develops, whereas what is not degenerates. He recommended frequent and varied exercise as the best preventive medicine. Romazzini, who was the author of the first book on occupational disease, published nearly 270 years ago, was convinced that a life lived mainly in a chair could lead only to a pallid complexion, poor physical condition, and, in general, poor health.

Both Hippocrates and Romazzini touched on a problem that to a great degree is magnified in today's society: The proliferation of labor-saving devices has allowed people to become physically passive. Only when the human motor fails—often as the result of self-imposed inactivity—do people begin to become aware of their own dwindling resources. What we call lifestyle diseases—coronary heart disease, digestive problems, the side-effects of obesity, certain forms of cancer, mental problems—cost society enormous sums of money each year. It is clear that preventive medicine must make far greater efforts to change people's health-destroying habits.

The effects of a sedentary life will eventually conquer the body. Muscles that are not in regular use, including the heart muscle, will weaken. The flexibility of the joints will be reduced. In weight-bearing joints, such as the hips and knees, the cartilage will become thinner and more vulnerable to overload and injury. Inactivity also causes the blood circulation in the muscular and skeletal structures to become less than efficient. Digestive problems, mental problems, weight problems, and all of the problems related to them can be aggravated or caused by physical inactivity.

This is quite a depressing run-down. But do not despair! Fortunately the human body is such a miraculous instrument that lost horsepower can generally be regained.

By now you should be well aware of the benefits of regular exercise. Physically, exercise strengthens the heart and other muscles, improves the circulation, increases lung capacity, and reduces the risk of cardiovascular and other diseases. Furthermore, physical well-being often means psychological well-being. Not only will exercise make you feel less tired, but your working capacity will actually increase. Stress and feelings of anxiety and tension can all be reduced or at least handled better if you are in good physical shape.

This chapter outlines a simple program of exercise, based on walking or jogging. You should use this to begin getting in shape very gradually, especially if years have passed since you last exercised regularly. For many, high school or college was the last time physical exercise was part of a daily routine. Once you are in shape, you can continue running, jogging, or walking, or substitute any aerobic exercise you prefer. Your goal should be to exercise the largest number of muscle groups and to give the most important muscle, the heart, a great deal of exercise. Bicycling, swimming, skiing, hiking, rowing, or other rhythmic activities will do this.

TESTING FITNESS LEVELS: THE STEP TEST.

To begin with, determine your present level of fitness. This can be done by arranging for a stress test on a treadmill or stationary bicycle at a sports clinic, under the guidance of professionals. Or you can get a rough idea of your fitness by putting yourself through a simple "step test."

Like other stress tests, the Step Test is strenuous, and unless you

Step up . . .

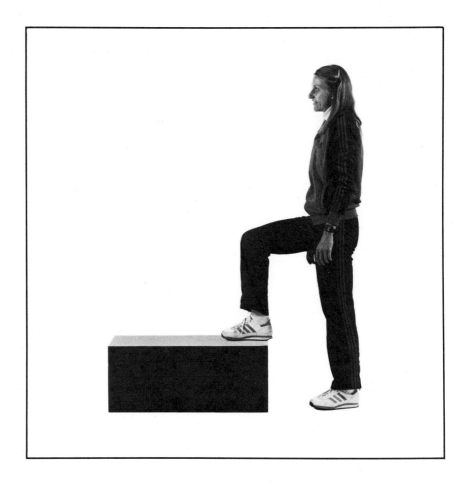

are in good general health and feel rested, you should not take it. Wear shorts, a light top, and light shoes. The test should be done in a relatively quiet, cool, well-ventilated but not drafty place. Aim for similar circumstances each time you test yourself. Before taking the test, you should wait for at least two hours after eating, and three hours if the meal was a heavy one. Persons who still smoke should wait at least two hours after having a cigarette.

Find a steady bench or stool that is approximately 19½ inches (50 cm) high for men and 15½ inches (40 cm) high for women. The height does not have to be exact, but it must be the same in each testing session. You will also need a watch with a second hand and, if possible, a metronome that can tick off 120 beats per minute. If you don't

. . . up.

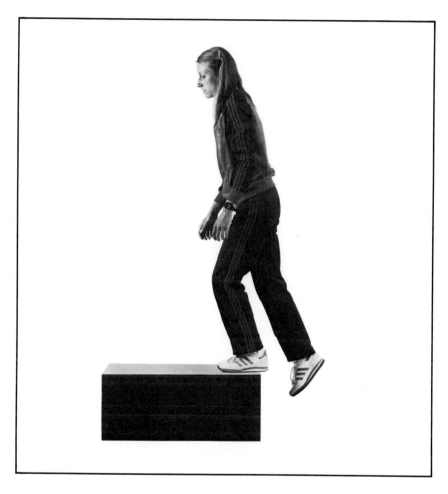

have a metronome, practice with the clock will help you to develop the proper rhythm.

The aim is to step up onto the bench, straighten your legs, then step back down off the bench, thirty times a minute, following the beats of the metronome—Left leg, Up! Right leg, Up! Left leg, Down! Right leg, Down! The same leg should lead each time you step onto the bench, although shifting legs once or twice during the test will not affect the results significantly.

If you fall out of rhythm because you become tired, stop. Take note of the time elapsed to the nearest fifth second and go on to the next part of the test. Otherwise, stop after five minutes.

Then down . . .

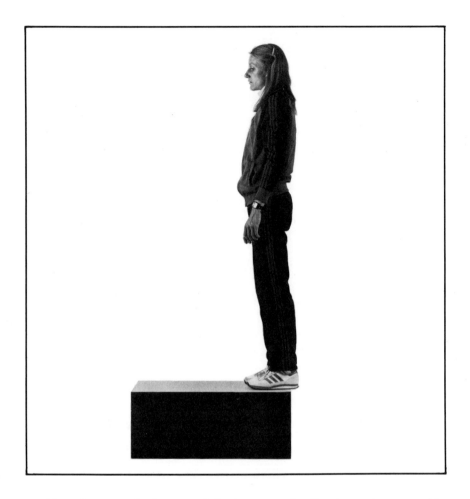

After the test, sit down and find your pulse (in the wrist or neck). Count the beats per thirty seconds as exactly as possible after one minute, after two minutes, and after four minutes. Be sure not to use your thumb to feel the pulse, since the pulse in the thumb itself will throw off your count. Compute the results of your test by multiplying the time in seconds by 100 and dividing this figure by twice the sum of the three pulse counts:

$$\text{Score:} \quad \frac{\text{Amount of time of test In seconds} \times 100}{\text{Total pulse count} \times 2}$$

Your fitness level is rated as follows:

Over 110 points	—very good
90–109	—good
70–89	—fair
55–69	—rather poor
Under 54	—poor

Take the test periodically to measure your fitness as it improves. Repeat it in exactly the same way each time. As you become more fit you will find that your pulse rate decreases, and you can use only the difference in pulse rates from one test to the next as an indicator of your progress.

The Step Test gives you a rough but adequate idea of your general fitness level. Other tests can also be used. One such test is the well-known Twelve-minute Running Test devised by Dr. Kenneth Cooper and described in his book *The Aerobics Way* (Bantam Books, 1971). Readers interested in having a more specific measure of their fitness than the one provided by the Step Test but who do not have access to a professional evaluation can put themselves through the paces of Dr. Cooper's test.

The Pulse Rate

To digress slightly, we should say a word about your pulse rate. As your heart muscle gets stronger it pumps more blood per heartbeat; the number of beats per minute (the pulse rate) is therefore reduced even when you are resting. Top athletes in endurance sports have been found to have a resting heartbeat as low as thirty beats per minute. However, this is unusual. At the other end of the spectrum, people in especially poor condition may have pulse rates as high as 90 to 100 beats a minute. The average range is 60 to 70 beats for men and 70 to 80 beats for women. The higher rate for women is caused by their somewhat lower concentration of red blood cells. This means that fewer "loads" of such cells—and therefore less of the oxygen that these cells carry—are dispatched per heartbeat, and the heart compensates with a slightly higher pumping rate (pulse).

. . . down.

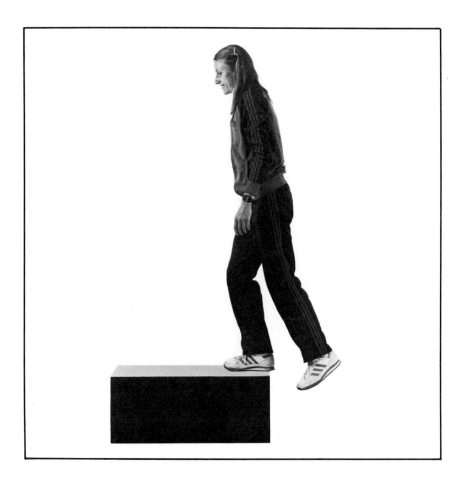

Although it can be considered a good indicator of training progress or regression, the resting pulse is affected by a number of different factors that somewhat lessen its value as an accurate measure of overall physical condition. Besides such factors as fatigue, eating, smoking, heat and humidity, the resting pulse is affected by colds, infections, and fever, as well as by emotional states. The position of the body also affects the resting pulse rate; the rate is highest when you are standing, somewhat lower when you are sitting, and lowest when you are lying down.

The best time to take your resting pulse is on waking in the morning. Find your pulse in your wrist or neck, count for fifteen seconds,

Achilles tendon, calf, and hamstring stretches. Keeping the back heel on the ground, extend your knee and stretch by pressing your hip forward. First stretch one leg, then the other. You can achieve a better stretching effect by placing the back foot farther away from your support.

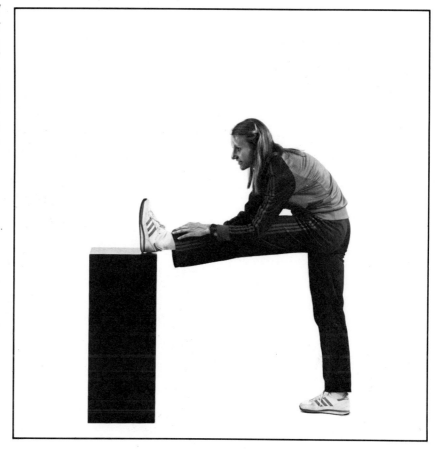

and multiply by four, or count for a full minute. Take your rate a couple of times for accuracy.

Training Intensity

To get the most out of the three-phase exercise program, the training should be strenuous enough to put your pulse rate within 70 to 85 percent of the maximal pulse rate.

The maximal pulse rate is the point at which the heart can no longer satisfy the body's demand for oxygen. It is the point at which you

You can also vary the stretching effect by stretching with your knee bent. Nearly the same effect will be achieved by placing your alternate heel up against the support. Keep your knee straight so that the front part of your foot is pointing upward. Stretch by pushing your hips toward the support.

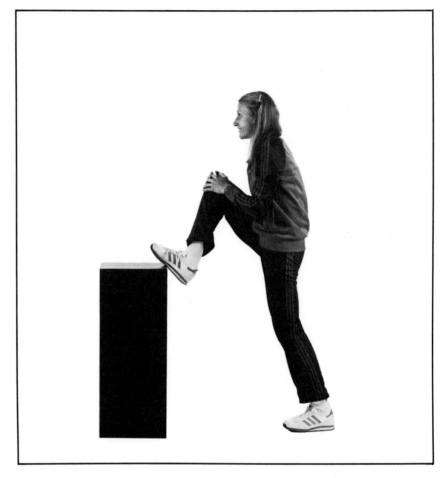

quickly become exhausted. The lower boundary of this intensity zone will allow you to carry on a conversation comfortably while training.

The maximal pulse rate is determined by subtracting your age from 220. For example, a forty-five-year-old will have a maximal pulse rate of 175 per minute, meaning an intensity zone during workouts of between 123 and 149 beats per minute (70 to 85 percent × 175). From the figure below, find the pulse-rate values that correspond to the upper and lower limits of your intensity zone.

Remember, your pulse may be affected by a number of different factors (see page 96); the pulse rate will be higher than normal during especially long training sessions when quite a bit of fluid is lost through sweating (and as the body temperature rises). The pulse rate also has a tendency to rise as one begins to tire. Therefore, the pulse rate as a training guide is most useful during short training sessions.

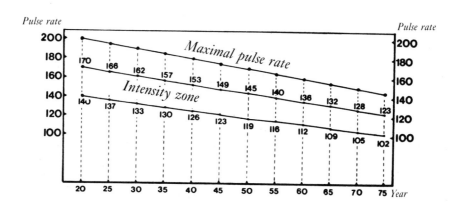

THE THREE-PHASE EXERCISE PROGRAM.

Every athlete in every sport follows the same three phases when training or competing: the warm-up phase, the exercise phase, and the cool-down or stretching phase.

Phase I: Warm Up

You are late and hurrying out of the house. As you approach the bus stop, a bus is just about to leave. You begin running as if the gun went off at a track meet. All goes well for a short distance and then your level of fitness is put to a rather uncomfortable test. Your breathing gets heavy, your heart pounds wildly, and your leg muscles ache. You sadly watch the bus disappear into the distance.

Almost everyone has had an experience like this at one time or another; the body simply fails to satisfy its sudden need for great quantities of oxygen. The price you pay is high: muscular stiffness and exhaustion. Warming up before you exert yourself may prevent this condition.

Oxygen is carried by the red blood cells from the lungs to the muscle cells through a dense web of capillaries. When you rest, the heart sends only about 15 percent of its blood output to the muscle mass. This amount increases to as much as 70 to 80 percent when your muscles are working hard. As this increase occurs, the body must ration the blood, reducing the blood supply to temporarily less important organ systems such as the digestive system, kidneys, and skin. Those organs that are working hard (the heart and muscles) have priority. Simultaneously, the nervous system acts on the muscles to open their blood vessels so that large quantities of blood can pass through the vessels and deliver oxygen and nutrition to the muscle cells. These adjustments do not happen instantaneously. It takes time to "tune" the body for exertion, and this tuning up is what we call the warm-up.

Your heart also needs a period of preparation for exercise. Blood flow through the heart increases considerably during heavy muscular work, and the heart must have enough time to adjust itself to this increased demand for blood. A study done in the United States a few years ago demonstrated the importance of such warming-up for the heart. A group of forty-four men were subjected to strenuous muscular activity of short duration both with and without prior warm-up sessions. They had to run up a steep hill on a treadmill at a speed of about 9.5 miles (15 kilometers) an hour. The heart's reaction to the overload was registered on an electrocardiogram (EKG), a graph that measures heart activity.

Prior to the experiment, the men were examined and none was found to have any signs of heart disease. The study showed that when they did not warm-up beforehand, 68 percent of the men had abnormal EKG results during their workout. On the other hand, when the men did warm-up exercises, such as jogging in place, before exercising, the abnormal EKG results were either reduced considerably or eliminated altogether. Furthermore, without prior warming up, the men's blood pressure was abnormally high both during and immediately following the workout, whereas with a prior warm-up it was greatly reduced. Warming up before exercising also lessens the chance of such injuries as pulled muscles and torn tendons.

Devise your own short program of ten to fifteen minutes of easy walking or jogging. Remember, you will *always* need to warm-up before exercising, regardless of the level of physical achievement you reach.

You can also use a sidewalk curb or a staircase landing (among other things) to achieve a good stretching effect for the Achilles tendon, calf, and hamstring. Stand with your heel hanging over the edge of the sidewalk and press down.

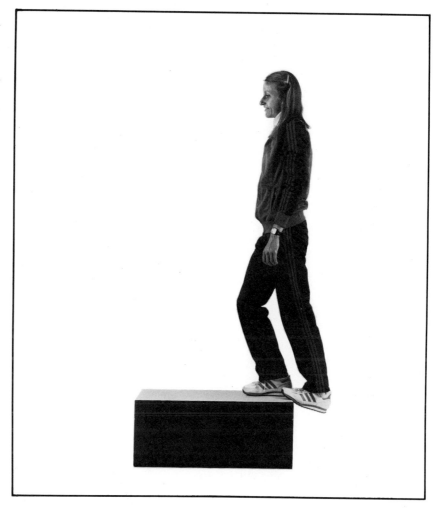

Phase II: Exercise

If minimal physical exertion, such as walking up the stairs, working in the garden, or carrying the groceries leaves you out of breath, you should start your training with a walking program. This will allow you to condition yourself to exercise gradually while at the same time avoiding injuries typical of those who start right in on a jogging/running program. After a long period of inactivity, the muscles, joints, tendons, and ligaments are especially sensitive to new demands and are easily hurt.

During the first few weeks, your training sessions should not last

Hamstring Stretch Two. Place your legs as shown. Bend the upper part of your body forward, keeping your back relatively straight and looking forward. Alternate legs. You can place your arms as shown in the figure or you can keep them behind your back.

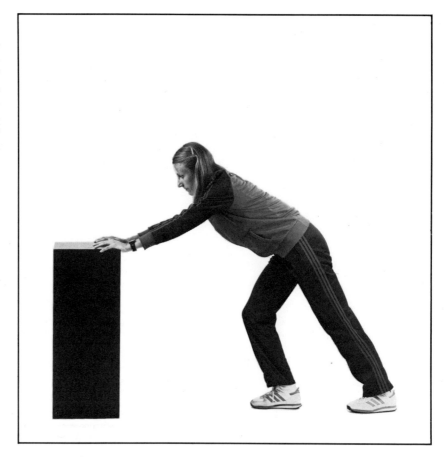

more than twenty to twenty-five minutes, including warm-up; the risk of injury increases considerably if training lasts much longer than this in the beginning. And you should train only two times a week during the first two or three weeks. By the fourth week you may exercise three times a week, and after the fifth week you may train every day if you wish. At that point, consider three days a minimum.

During this transition period, do not be tempted to begin jogging or running. You will be increasing the pressure on your ankle, knee, and hip joints by two or three times, and will only be risking injury.

After the first few weeks of training you will begin feeling your body getting into shape. Start making slightly greater demands on the

Additional hamstring stretch can be achieved by pressing the toes against a support, alternating legs, and keeping the heel of both the front and back foot down.

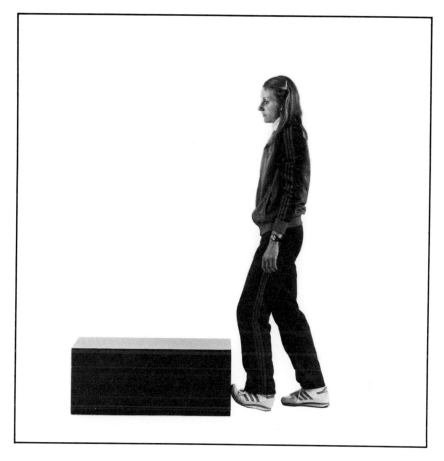

heart and circulatory system by increasing your walking pace and including more hills in your route. Try varying the terrain—the edges of fields, forest paths, marshy areas, or soft, sandy beaches. The softer surfaces require an extra expenditure of energy.

After about six weeks you will feel noticeably more energetic. You will then be ready to take on new challenges, and you should start a jogging/walking program as explained below. Jogging and running put even greater demands on the heart and circulation, which gradually adjust to the higher workload, thus becoming stronger and more efficient.

At first, do not jog for more than a few minutes (five at most) at a

Calf and thigh stretch. Hold one foot as shown. You may want to use only one hand. Stand with your body erect and pull your foot up, pressing your heel in toward your body.

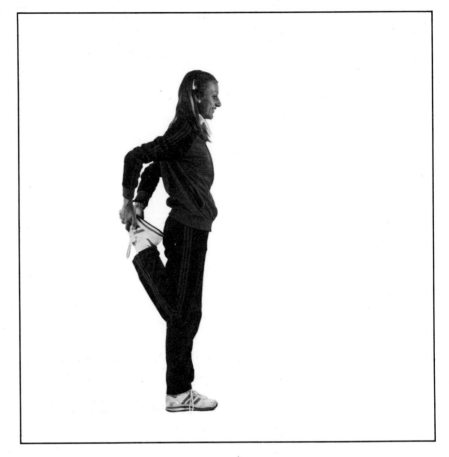

time, and always start with walking and brisk walking until you have warmed up thoroughly. Then jog slowly for a while, go back to walking, and then jog again. Alternate in this way between jogging and walking for ten to fifteen minutes.

Remember that the pressure on your ankle, knee, and hip joints is especially great while jogging and running downhill. Those who are overweight are especially vulnerable to injuries of these joints and should keep to relatively flat terrain in the beginning. Look for soft surfaces—tracks and grassy fields—and always wear well-cushioned running shoes.

Gradually, as you get stronger, you can increase the time you run

Hip joints. Assume the position shown. Stretch your back foot out and push your hip area down. Alternate between legs.

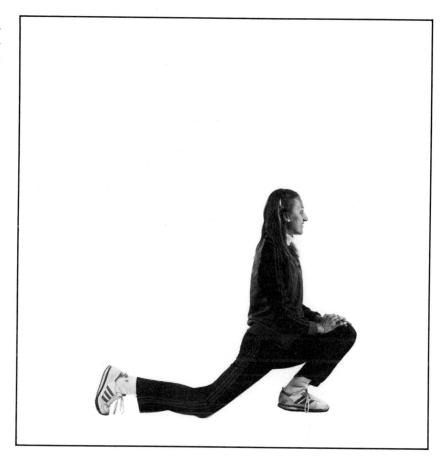

and decrease the time you walk until, if you wish, you are jogging and running for the entire twenty-five minutes, beginning with fifteen minutes of slow jogging.

Phase III: Cool-Down

When muscles and joints are put through a repetitive and limited range of motion, as in jogging, running, and bicycling, they may gradually lose their flexibility. To prevent this, all athletes—at every level—perform regular stretching exercises after training. This restores and maintains a minimum degree of flexibility, which allows unrestricted movements and provides resistance to injury.

When you have finished exercising, stretch your muscles slowly and gradually and do not overextend them. Maintain a stretched position for ten to fifteen seconds and concentrate on releasing all tension from your body. Repeat this several times. When you become accustomed to the exercises, the stretching time may be increased to twenty to thirty seconds or even longer. If time permits, also stretch parts of the body not used during your exercises. Avoid or be careful with stretching exercises that produce pain in the joints or lower back. If you are in doubt about any such exercise, drop it until you have consulted an expert. The exercises shown are especially suited to jogging, running, and walking.

IN SHAPE AFTER FIFTY.

"Sports—all the training, competitions, and excitement—has created a kind of need in me. There is simply nothing like the feeling of well-being that envelops me after a good physical workout." This comment, made by an over-fifty athlete, is typical of people who have kept in good condition during the years. They reach their retirement with a biological age of much younger individuals.

When you are young and exercise is almost an automatic part of your daily regimen, your level of physical fitness develops relatively quickly. This level stabilizes in the mid-twenties and, with regular training, remains more or less unchanged through the thirties. As part of the aging process, a gradual decline in the heart's pumping capacity then takes place. This is due to a reduced maximal pulse rate as well as a weakening in the strength of the heart's contractions. The capacity of the heart to fill with blood may also be reduced.

Major changes in one's activity level will also change one's level of physical fitness immediately and often dramatically; for example, three weeks of lying in bed will lead to a 30 percent reduction in the physical-fitness level. The combination of physical inactivity and aging will turn normal daily activities into heavy work relatively quickly. The gradual weight gain of many elderly people further contributes to a reduced work capacity.

Aging should not, however, stop you from getting into shape. The human body remains responsive to physical training well into the seventies and eighties. There are numerous examples of older people doing physical activities normally associated only with the young. Larry Lewis, who died in 1974 at the age of 106, took his daily run of six miles around the borders of Golden Gate Park in San Francisco right to the end of his life—and did this before he went to his work as a waiter in a hotel. His response to the many drivers who offered him a lift was a polite, "No, thank you. My legs were made for use, not misuse."

"I will run until I am one hundred years old," said the Norwegian Georg B. Vang after he, at the age of seventy, placed second in the Veteran Championship marathon (26.2 miles) with a finishing time of four hours and one minute. At the age of eighty, Vang still trains almost every day. "It is so good to feel healthy, and for this I have my regular year-round training program to thank," he says. He began training at the age of fifty-three with the walk/run program. After only six months, he ran 5,000 meters (3.1 miles) in twenty-two and a half minutes. In his mid-sixties he dreamed of participating in a marathon and increased the intensity of his training. At the age of sixty-seven he completed his first marathon in an impressive three hours, twenty-one minutes, and twenty-nine seconds.

A look at the result from the 1979 New York marathon shows that age is not necesarily a handicap in competing with the best runners. For example, Piet Van Alpen of Holland (age forty-nine) finished in 2:30:13. Others included Ron Hill (age forty-two), of England, 2:23:20; and the American Fritz Mueller (age forty-three), 2:27:55. Forty-four-year-old Maria D'Orlando of Italy took sixteenth place among the women, finishing in under three hours.

The following figure shows that sudden inactivity causes a rapid drop in the physical fitness level (upper left corner). It also demonstrates that a thirty-year-old, by beginning a regular exercise program, can actively prevent further loss in physical fitness, and in fact raise the fitness level in his or her forties and fifties.

Physical fitness level (given as aerobic power)

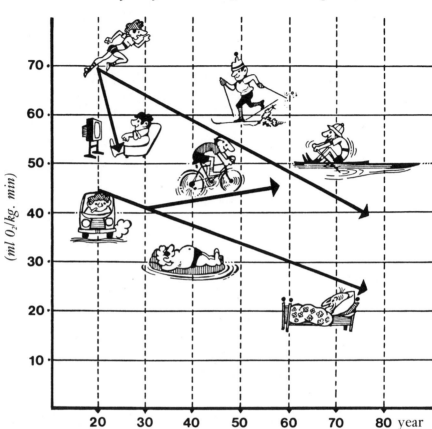

But what about people who are older when they *start* training? In one study, a group of people whose average age was seventy (the oldest was seventy-eight) trained on a stationary bicycle three times a week for three months, doing interval workouts lasting from six to ten minutes. The program resulted in an approximate 38 percent increase in the subjects' physical fitness level. It is never too late to begin!

The training program for persons over fifty is essentially the same as for everyone else. It follows the three phases: warm-up, exercise, and cool-down. The difference is that the program should be followed more slowly and the training intensity increased more gradually. It is never necessary to exhaust yourself to get into shape. It is generally better to have longer training sessions of moderate intensity than to train more intensively over short periods. From the figure on page 99 and the accompanying text, you will be able to see how your pulse rate can be used as a training guide.

Older people will also need a longer period of recuperation after each training session. Therefore, see to it that your body gets adequate rest between training sessions. For many, this means exercising no more than every other day. There is, however, considerable individual variation in the reaction to training, and some people may be able to exercise more frequently than this.

THE MOVE TO LOSE WEIGHT.

As many as one-third of all people are overweight. Although the causes of excess body weight may be quite complex, in most cases such excess is due to nothing more than a combination of physical inactivity and overeating; In only a very few cases can excessive weight be blamed on a faulty metabolism. However, hereditary factors do play a role in determining body weight. The number of fat cells as well as the resting metabolic rate can vary considerably from individual to individual. And, although overeating probably does not increase the number of fat cells, it may increase the size of the individual fat cells almost without limit.

Excess weight and obesity are not always the same thing. Your weight depends on your bone structure and muscle development. A person with a well-trained and developed body may, for example, weigh much more than any of the height/weight charts you might have seen in various diet books. The ultimate test of whether or not you are overweight is simply to look in the mirror.

As simple as it sounds, most people can control their body weight through a combined program of regular exercise and proper eating. Forget about all the fad diets, about replacing delicious food with pills, powders, glasses of water, and other such things. The simple fact is that as long as your energy supply does not exceed your energy demand, excessive weight will not be a problem. In other words, do not eat more food than your body will need.

In beginning to lose weight, your food choices should be low-calorie, with a total intake of from 1,100 to 1,500 kilocalories per day. Your weight loss should be gradual. You should not try to lose more than about a pound (0.5 kilogram) per week. In three months time, this means a loss of about twelve pounds (5.5 kilos) of fat. Such a weight-loss program involves a daily reduction of about 500 kilocalories, and this is certainly easy to maintain if you follow the advice we give below. A slight feeling of hunger and a few self-denials are a small price to pay for the satisfaction of reaching your goal.

Experience shows that you will be much better off if you can diet along with someone you know. Devise a plan you will both follow—get together frequently, encourage each other.

PRACTICAL HINTS FOR LOSING WEIGHT

- Cut down a little on the amount of food you take at each meal.
- Substitute whole-grain breads and other grain products, vegetables, and fruits for fatty meats and other high-fat foods.
- Avoid french fries, potato chips, peanuts, chocolate, sugar candy, and other foods high in fat or sugar.
- Avoid or cut down on the use of sugar and cream in your coffee and tea.
- Drink skimmed milk instead of whole milk.
- Use light margarine or nothing at all.
- Use light mayonnaise and other light dressings. Better still, do not use any dressing.
- Trim any excess fat from meat, and do not add fat as you cook.
- Chew your food well and drink plenty of water.
- Do not eat between meals.
- To curb your appetite before dinner, you should eat a carrot or apple. You will then eat less at the dinner table.

To lose and then maintain your reduced weight, exercise regularly, three times a week. It is best to do thirty to sixty minutes of aerobic

ACTIVITY	KCAL/MIN	KCAL/HR	KJ/MIN	MJ/HR
Walking on flat ground at a speed of				
2.5m/hr(4km/hr)	4	240	17	1.0
3.1m/hr(5km/hr)	5	300	21	1.3
3.7m/hr(6km/hr)	6	360	25	1.5
4.3m/hr(7km/hr)	7	420	29	1.8
Jogging at				
5m/hr(8km/hr)	10	600	42	2.5
6.2m/hr(10km/hr)	11	660	46	2.8
Running at				
7.5m/hr(12km/hr)	15	900	63	3.8
7.3m/hr(15km/hr)	18	1080	76	4.5
Cycling at				
3.7m/hr(22km/hr)	10	600	42	2.5
Tennis	5–10	300–600	21–42	1.3–2.5
Skiing	10–20	600–1200	42–84	2.5–5.0
Soccer	7–10	420–600	29–42	1.8–2.5
Swimming	5–11	300–660	21–46	1.3–2.8
Cutting grass	5–8	300–480	21–34	1.3–2.0

activity such as jogging or running, bicycling, skiing, swimming, playing certain ball games, and modern or jazz dancing. But remember to go very slowly in the beginning. An overweight body needs more time than a normal one to adjust to the extra demands of exercise. Follow the three-phase exercise plan and be certain to keep the intensity within your range. Either take your pulse at intervals or try the talk test. Exercise burns up calories. The chart below will give you a rough estimate of the calorie consumption in various types of activities.

Look for ways to add more exercise to your daily routine. Walk to and from work, for example, and begin using the stairs instead of the elevator. You will burn even more calories.

Mental training along with exercise and a proper diet will help you through the slow, often frustrating process of losing weight. Devise your own Training Sequences according to your own diet problems, and practice them daily.

As exercise and training become more and more an integral part of your weekly routine, you may very well begin looking forward to training sessions as much as to a good meal. In other words, your appetite for exercise increases! When this happens, you know for sure that the battle of the bulge is won.

TRAINING SEQUENCE FOR WEIGHT REDUCTION

I can achieve my goal of weight reduction.
I will control myself and resist temptations.
I will make my own decisions to reduce my weight.
I have sufficient willpower to reduce my weight.
I will choose the right foods.
Losing weight will be good for me.

9 Training for Competition

Many people who exercise regularly sooner or later develop the desire to test their strength. Others compete simply for the camaraderie of competitive sports. And the sport that has become most popular and accessible almost everywhere in the world is running. Joggers become runners, become racers. It takes only a pair of running shoes, a small entry fee, and adequate training to enable you to toe the starting line with the world's most elite runners.

The running boom is most evident in the United States. In 1970, the first New York City marathon had a field of 126 runners. Just a decade later, the race, run through the city streets, had swelled its ranks to 14,012 marathoners, with many thousands more turned away for lack of space. But not everyone will feel the lure of the 26.2-mile marathon. Shorter races and "fun runs" are becoming increasingly popular. People of all ages and abilities run the course and receive certificates for finishing, not winning. Success and improvement are individual targets, and this is encouraging to runners with limited time or motivation to race.

Any race requires preparation. During competition, the demands on the body are great and can be met only if you have followed a well-planned training program and are aware of the body's response to hard physical strain and such external factors as extreme heat and cold. This practical information can be crucial in determining how well you perform in competitions.

Essentially, the body needs to develop endurance and speed for distance races. While there are many methods for doing this, the most common are long, slow distance running for endurance and interval training for speed.

LONG, SLOW DISTANCE TRAINING.

This method is based on the principle of continuity. Endurance is developed by running at a slow, steady pace over a long period of time. As the body adapts, it becomes better able to tolerate the prolonged heavy workloads involved in such exercise. The length of time spent on this type of training depends on one's physical condition. It is best to begin with a minimum of twenty minutes of slow running and to gradually increase the time to an hour or more. Some runners regularly schedule a three-hour long, slow distance run in their weekly routine.

Remember to keep the intensity of your training at a low level. If you can carry on a conversation relatively easily while running, you are running at the right pace.

INTERVAL TRAINING.

This method is slightly more complicated than long, slow distance running. You will alternate between resting and working, between high and low intensity during your workout.

Natural Interval

With natural-interval training, the terrain over which you train determines the intensity and duration of your workout interval. Hills and soft surfaces such as sand, for example, offer resistance and require extra effort. Include sections of varying terrain in your course, and try to maintain an even and relatively high intensity in uphill sections or when going through sand. Do not allow your muscles to stiffen, however. Run the same natural-interval training routes several times a week and compare your running times. The duration of your running should be from thirty minutes to two hours.

Fartlek ("playing with speed")

As its name implies, you should have fun with this method. *Fartlek* allows you to improvise with your running, alternating between high and low intensity. In the course of your running sprint every so often, or take on a very tough hill—a sand dune if you can find one. Although *fartlek* is more or less unsystematic, it should include a certain degree of planning and order, and you should work hard for a least half of your workout, allowing plenty of rest time between intense intervals. Vary the time, terrain, length of your stride, and speed.

Short Interval

This type of training involves relatively short work periods that alternate with short rest periods. For most runners, this means work periods of two minutes and rest periods of about thirty seconds—so short that the oxygen intake and thus the pulse rate drops very little before the next work period begins.

Short-interval training forces you to have maximal or near maximal oxygen intake. This does not necessarily mean that you must work at maximal intensity; the goal is to adjust the intensity of your exercise during the work periods to bring you close to your maximal oxygen intake without causing muscle stiffness. Active rest periods are the most effective means for achieving this, and you should jog slowly during these pauses.

Long Interval

The work periods in long-interval training range from two to ten minutes, with rest periods of two to five minutes to allow you to work equally hard during each work period.

Your training intensity should be so high that your pulse rate is a mere twenty beats under your maximal pulse rate per minute. Persons in good condition can work at an even higher intensity.

Long-interval training can be quite demanding, and should not be attempted until you have a good training background. Begin carefully with short periods of work and slowly increase the length of the work periods, gradually increasing your training load by shortening the pauses between workouts. The number of work-period repetitions usually varies between two and ten.

TRAINING SCHEDULES.

No matter what your racing goals, you should formulate a training schedule not only to assure adequate preparation but to be at peak level on the day of a race. Below are training schedules for runners at varying levels and for races of varying distances.

The Occasional Racer

This four-day-a-week schedule will prepare you for any middle distance race under 10 kilometers (6.2 miles). The week before the race, you should drop one "hard" day and, if you want to run three times a week, drop day 3.

DAY

1.	Easy	Long, slow distance training: 4 to 6 miles (6.4 to 9.7 kilometers) of easy running.
2.	Hard	*Fartlek* about thirty to thirty-five minutes; long-distance training with increased speed over short distances (from 150 to 600 yards, or 137 to 549 meters). Try to do about six or seven sprints.
3.	Easy	Long, slow distance training: 6 to 8 miles (9.7 to 12.9 kilometers) of easy running.
4.	Easy/ Hard	Slow distance training 2 to 3 miles (3.2 to 4.8 kilometers), then fast distance training for the same distance. Finish the session with a half mile of easy jogging.

Competitive Runners

This is a regular schedule to follow for maintaining a good training base. If you are aiming for a specific 10-kilometer race or a marathon, you can easily shift over from this schedule to one of the schedules shown in the boxes on pp. 119–122.

Drop day 1 or 5 if you want to keep your training to four days a week. For a three-day week use either the days 1-2-3 or the days 1-3-4 schedule. If there is a race day coming up at the end of the week, drop one hard training day and maybe one easy one. If the race is very important to you, train easily the entire week before it.

Ten-Kilometer Race

This schedule is set up for those with a race goal of one hour or less. You should plan on training three times a week (Monday, Wednesday, and Friday; or Tuesday, Thursday, and Saturday), and should count on at least ten weeks of preparation. The chart gives you a program for the first five weeks; after this you should be able to design the rest of the training program to suit your needs.

You must have a good training base before you begin to race. Spend at least six months on the three-phase walk/jog/run program described in Chapter 8.

Run at the pace that you find comfortable and adjust your schedule accordingly. Your further progress should be based on this pace. For example, if you find that five-and-a-half minutes per kilometer (instead of six or seven minutes as suggested in the program) is a comfortable pace, start at this tempo and adjust the rest of the program so that you have a reasonable increase in workload from week to week.

Remember to use at least the first mile of jogging to warm up. One day a week of interval training will increase your speed and be especially beneficial to the cardiovascular system. The pace of your interval-training sprints should be adjusted according to your own fitness level; but remember, never run so fast that you begin to notice stiffening of your leg muscles.

Try to include some hilly terrain in your route. Running uphill at an even speed will automatically require an extra effort and will strengthen you.

After five weeks, your workouts should last for sixty to seventy minutes, and the distance should be increased to a total of 6 to 8 miles (9.7 to 12.9 kilometers). Try to add a longer training run one day a week, at an easy pace. It is also important to schedule a rest day of easy effort after every hard day of training.

DAY

1.	Easy/ Hard	Long-distance training: 5 miles (8 kilometers)—10 miles (16 kilometers) of easy running, 4 miles (6.4 kilometers) at close to racing pace, and 1 mile (1.6 kilometers) of jogging.
2.	Hard	Interval training after 1½ miles (2.4 kilometers) of slow jogging. Sprint for 300 yards (274 meters), with a one-minute rest break (you can run on a track or on grass, roads, or dirt). Repeat this ten times. Finish with 1 mile (1.6 kilometers) of easy running.
3.	Easy	Long, slow distance training: 8 to 10 miles (12.9 to 16 kilometers) or more.
4.	Hard	*Fartlek*, forty-five minutes: increase the speed over short distances (200 to 1,000 yards or 183 to 914 kilometers. Try to do about ten such sprints.
5.	Easy	Long, slow distance training: about 7 to 10 miles (11.2 to 16 kilometers).

Marathon Training for Beginners

The 26.2-mile marathon distance demands an exceptionally strong training base, not only to permit completing the marathon, but in order to avoid injury. To run continually for three to four hours on a hard surface is extremely stressful to muscles, bones, joints, ligaments, and tendons. Many people have been injured by learning this the hard way, and as a result have been forced to stop running altogether until they recover.

WEEK	1st DAY	Dist km	/ mi	Time min	2nd DAY	Dist km	/ mi	Time min	3rd DAY	Dist km	/ mi	Time min
1	Jog	2	1.2	15–16	Jog	2	1.2	15–16	Jog	2	1.2	15–16
	Run	1	0.6	6–7	Run	1	0.6	6–7	Run	2	1.2	13–14
	Walk	1	0.6	9–10	Walk	1	0.6	9–10	Walk	1	0.6	9–10
	Jog	1	0.6	7–8	Jog	1	0.6	7–8	Jog	1	0.6	7–8
Total		5	3.1	37–41		5	3.1	37–41		6	3.7	44–48
2	Jog	2	1.2	15–16	Jog	2	1.2	15–16	Jog	2	1.2	15–16
	Run	1	0.6	6–7	Run	4×.02	(4×0.12)	Time pr 200m <1 min. Pause 2 min. Equals approx 10 min.	Run	2	1.2	14–15
	Walk	1	0.6	9	Jog	1	0.6	7–8	Jog	2	1.2	15–16
	Run	1	0.6	6–7	Run	2	1.2	13–14	Run	1	0.6	6–7
	Jog	1	0.6	7–8	Walk	1	0.6	9	Walk	1	0.6	9
Total		6	3.7	44–47		6.8	4.2	54–57		8	5	59–63

The training schedule below is based on a long, slow process of building up your physical conditioning to marathon level. It stretches over a six-month period, and each four-week cycle is based on the progression: easy week, moderate week, hard week, easy week. The total distance increases slowly from 15 to 40 miles (24 to 64 kilometers) per week. The longest distance in one workout is 16 miles (26 kilometers). It is *not* necessary to run the full marathon distance during training. It is also important to ease up during the last ten to fourteen days before the marathon. Your last long run of 16 miles should be taken before this time. In the final week before the marathon, concentrate on diet and nutrition rather than training. Finally, get used to drinking water regularly during your training sessions, since you will need to drink while running the marathon.

PRERACE WARM-UP.

It is even more important to stretch and warm up before a race than

WEEK		1st DAY				2nd DAY				3rd DAY		
		Dist km / mi		Time min		Dist km / mi		Time min		Dist km / mi		Time min
	Jog	2	1.2	14–15	Jog	2	1.2	14–15	Jog	3	1.9	22–23
	Run	1	0.6	6–7	Run	5×0.2	(5×0.12)	Time pr 200m <1 min. Pause 1 min. Equals approx 10 min.	Run	2	1.2	14–15
3												
	Jog	1	0.6	7–8	Jog	1	0.6	7–8	Jog	1½	0.9	11–12
	Run	1	0.6	6–7	Run	2	1.2	13–14	Run	1	0.6	6–7
	Jog	2	1.2	15–16	Jog	1	0.6	7–8	Jog	1	0.6	7–8
Total		7	4.3	48–53		7	4.3	51–55		8½	5.3	60–65

before a training run. The general rule is that the shorter the racing distance, the more thoroughly you need to warm up; it takes about twenty minutes of activity before you begin to work at peak capacity, and you would not want to waste the first part of a short race just warming up.

WEEK	1st DAY			2nd DAY			3rd DAY		
		Dist km / mi	Time min		Dist km / mi	Time min		Dist km / mi	Time min
4	Jog	3	1.9	21–22	Jog	3	1.9	21–22	Jog	3	1.9	21–22
	Run	1	0.6	5–6	Run	6×0.2	(6×0.12)	Time pr 200m <1 min. Pause 1 min. Equals approx 12 min.	Run	2	1.2	13–14
	Jog	1	0.6	7–8	Jog	1	0.6	7–8	Jog	2	1.2	15–16
	Run	1	0.6	5–6	Run	2	1.2	13–14	Run	1	0.6	6–7
	Jog	2	1.2	14–15	Jog	1	0.6	7–8	Jog	1	0.6	7–8
Total		8	5.0	52–57		8.2	5.1	60–64		9	5.6	62–67
5	Jog	3	4.9	21–22	Jog	3	4.9	21–22	Jog	3	4.9	21–22
	Run	2	1.2	12–13	Run	3×0.3	(3×0.19)	Time pr 300m <1½ min. Pause 1½ min. Equals approx 9 min.	Run	3	4.9	19–20
	Jog	2	1.2	14–15	Jog	2	1.2	15–16	Jog	2	1.2	14–15
	Run	1	0.6	5–6	Run	1	0.6	5–6	Run	1	0.6	6–7
	Jog	2	1.2	14–15	Jog	3	4.9	21–22	Jog	1	0.6	7–8
Total		10	6.2	66–71		9.9	6.2	71–75		10	6.2	67–72

For longer races, such as marathons, there is no need for a lengthy pre-race warm-up phase. Instead, it is good race strategy to include a warm-up period in the race itself by beginning at a moderate speed for

DISTANCE PER DAY IN KILOMETERS/MILES

WEEK	1st DAY		2nd DAY		3rd DAY		4th DAY		TOTAL DISTANCE PER WEEK
E.G.→	MONDAY		TUESDAY		THURSDAY		SATURDAY		
	KM	MI	KM	MI	KM	MI	KM	MI	
1	6	3.7	5	3.1	10	6.2	4	2.5	25	15.5
2	7	4.3	6	3.7	11	6.8	5	3.1	29	18
3	8	5	7	4.3	14	8.7	6	3.7	35	21.7
4	6	3.7	5	3.1	10	6.2	4	2.5	25	15.5
5	8	5	7	4.3	12	7.5	6	3.7	33	20.5
6	9	5.6	8	5	13	8.1	7	4.3	37	23
7	10	6.2	9	5.6	16	9.9	8	5	43	26.7
8	8	5.9	7	4.3	12	7.5	6	3.7	33	20.5
9	10	6.2	9	5.6	14	8.7	8	5	41	25.5
10	11	6.8	10	6.2	15	9.3	9	5.6	45	28
11	12	7.5	11	6.8	20	12.4	10	6.2	53	32.9
12	10	6.2	9	5.6	14	8.7	8	5	41	25.5
13	12	7.5	11	6.8	16	9.9	10	6.2	49	30.4
14	13	8.1	12	7.5	17	10.6	11	6.8	53	32.9
15	14	8.7	13	8.1	22	35.4	12	7.5	61	37.9
16	12	7.5	11	6.8	16	9.9	10	6.2	49	30.4
17	14	8.7	13	8.1	18	11.2	12	7.5	57	35.4
18	15	9.3	14	8.7	19	11.8	13	8.1	61	37.9
19	16	9.9	15	9.3	24	14.9	14	8.7	69	42.9
20	14	8.7	13	8.1	18	11.2	12	7.5	57	37.9
21	16	9.9	15	9.3	20	12.4	14	8.7	65	40.4
22	17	10.6	16	9.9	21	13	15	9.3	69	42.9
23	18	11.2	17	10.6	26	16.2	16	9.9	77	47.8
24	16	9.9	15	9.3	20	12.4	14	8.7	65	40.4

the first few miles. A slow start will often leave you with enough energy to speed up in the last few miles, and you will frequently find that you catch up with and pass those who started fast and have worn themselves out.

At the start of almost every race, the air is filled with the characteristic aroma of "deep-heating" salves, which some runners rub into their limbs in the mistaken belief that these preparations will directly help to warm up their muscles. The salves do create a feeling of warmth and a reddening of the skin, but this is because they dilate the capillaries of the skin. If anything, the salves will increase the difference in temperature between the skin and the air, increasing the loss of heat from the body; they have no real effect on the temperature of the muscles, and are therefore useless as far as performance goes. Save your money.

Another pointless warm-up practice is taking a hot shower, bath, or sauna before a race. This *will* cause the body temperature to rise, and in an attempt to keep the temperature at 98.6°F, the body will send blood rushing to the outer layers of the skin. The blood circulation in the muscles, however, does not change noticeably.

PRERACE GUIDELINES

Do stretch and warm up before every race.
Do warm up longer before shorter races.
Do start a long race at a slow pace.
Do drink some water before a long race.
Don't substitute "deep-heat" salves for warm-up exercises.
Don't warm up by raising your body temperature with a bath or shower.

FOOD FOR RACING.

Nutritional deposits in the body and their ready availability will affect your performance on the day of a race. The body's main sources of energy are carbohydrates and fat. Carbohydrates, the runner's preferred fuel, are stored mainly as glycogen—a starch-like substance—in the muscles and liver. There is much less glycogen than fat in the body, and when during a long race the supply runs out, a collapse occurs. This is the phenomenon known as "hitting the wall." In a marathon it most frequently occurs at the 20-mile (32-kilometer) point. The body becomes sluggish, the blood sugar level is low, and coordination, reaction speed, and concentration are lost.

Glycogen depletion cannot always be prevented, but there are several things you can do to avoid it. First, race at your own level of physical fitness, and do not keep pace with those who are in better condition. Also, do not start off too hard; in such cases, the expenditure of glycogen in the first few miles will be especially high. Moreover, an intense early pace, especially for a beginner, usually means that the muscles will need more oxygen than the body can supply. Lactic acid then builds up in the muscle cells, causing muscle stiffness and the inhibition of the body's ability to use fat as fuel.

Well-trained athletes with plenty of race experience seldom hit the wall. Their regular endurance training ensures an increased ability to mobilize fat from the places in the body where it is stored, and a greater capacity of the muscle cells to use fat as fuel. In other words, regular endurance training permits the body to use fat, of which it has a good supply, and to economize on glycogen, which is scarcer, during prolonged physical exertion. It also appears that physical training improves the ability of the liver to produce sugar from fat and protein.

For most runners, a sensible, well-balanced diet combined with adequate training and rest, as well as realistic race goals, will produce a satisfying race effort. Many runners, however, do feel that their performance is improved by a diet regimen known as carbohydrate loading. This regimen should be followed only before a race of marathon distance or longer. Its purpose is to increase the amount of glycogen in the body by carefully increasing the amount of carbohydrate in the diet.

If you wish to use carbohydrate loading, take a long slow run, a week before the race, to deplete your glycogen supply, and begin a three-day program of moderate workouts combined with low-carbohydrate foods. On the fourth day, begin three days of rest and carbohydrate-rich foods—at least 75 percent of your daily calorie allowance should be coming from the carbohydrate food group. This does *not* mean that you should be overeating; only that carbohydrates should make up most of your meals.

CARBOHYDRATE-LOADING DIET

DAY	PLAN
1–3	Depletion phase. Choose foods low in carbohydrates: fish, beef, pork, green vegetables, tomatoes, water. Avoid coffee, tea, beer, sugar, bread.
4–6	Loading phase. Choose foods high in carbohydrates: whole grain breads, potatoes, cereals, rice, pasta, fresh and dried fruits, ice cream, cakes.
7	Continue carbohydrate-rich diet at breakfast and lunch. Eat a light evening meal.
8	Race day.

This diet plan is still a controversial one. It is not guaranteed to give you a better race performance, nor does it seem to work for every runner or on every race occasion. There are too many variables, and test results with the diet have been inconsistent. The depletion phase is unpleasant at best, and many runners would be better off following a regular, balanced diet or a modified plan with two days of depletion and three days of loading.

At almost every starting line you will see some runners gobbling handfuls of carbohydrate-rich snacks—everything from chocolate to gumdrops—in the hope that these sugary foods will give them instant energy. High-sugar foods can cause a greatly increased secretion of the hormone insulin (which removes sugar from the blood) and thus a parallel decrease in the blood sugar level after about twenty minutes of running. You will feel weak and sluggish instead of energetic.

Another dubious practice is dosing yourself with large quantities of vitamins. The body will simply rid itself of any surplus water-soluble vitamins, such as the B vitamins and vitamin C. However, other vitamins—notably vitamins A and D—are stored in the body, and can be harmful when taken in overdoses.

"Shock doses" of vitamin C, although often suggested for colds, should also be avoided. Vitamin C is an acid and, taken in excess, is flushed from the body through the urinary tract. Eventually, it may cause kidney stones to develop, especially if you also drink relatively small quantities of water and other fluids. It also causes flatulence and, in some people, diarrhea—conditions uncomfortable at all times and intolerable when one is competing.

A well-balanced diet, rather than vitamin supplements, will meet any suddenly increased bodily demand for vitamins. However, if you feel that your diet may be vitamin deficient, you should certainly take a daily vitamin supplement, following the directions on the package.

KEEPING COOL.

Heat is the runner's archenemy. Hot, humid weather inhibits the effectiveness of the body's natural cooling system. Sweat, instead of evaporating quickly and thus cooling the skin, sits on the surface, drenching but not cooling. The body temperature rises, and for runners this means danger.

In its effort to maintain its proper temperature, the body sweats a great deal. In hot weather, and with exercise, this can easily lead to a significant loss of body fluid, and without adequate replacement of this fluid, the cooling mechanism is further weakened. Heat exhaustion or heat-stroke then become threats. Heat-stroke can cause permanent damage or death. Every summer the various publications devoted to running warn against the dangers of overexertion in hot weather, and almost every year there are stories of tragedies—of runners who were unaware of the dangers or ignored the symptoms of heat-stroke. Do not be a statistic; learn to recognize both the dangers and the symptoms of this condition.

Heat Exhaustion

If the amount of heat produced during running, especially in hot weather, is larger than the amount of heat the body gives off, the runner's body temperature will rise above what is normal increase during muscular work. This high temperature disturbs several important body functions; the runner will feel weak and uncomfortable, experiencing varying degrees of dizziness, headache, nausea, sleepiness, and weakening of eyesight. This condition is called *heat exhaustion*.

As soon as you feel any of these symptoms during a run or race, stop running! Find a shady, preferably cool place and begin to cool down. Douse your body and drink cold water. Get help. Heat exhaustion can easily escalate into the more dangerous condition known as *heat-stroke*.

Heat-stroke

This is the most serious and dangerous condition resulting from heat stress. The transition from heat exhaustion to stroke is very subtle. It can come on suddenly and without warning.

Heat-stroke causes unconsciousness (fainting); delirium (confusion, hallucinations); rapid, difficult breathing; dry, reddish, and hot skin (discontinued sweating); choking; and vomiting. A few or all of these symptoms may occur in varying degrees. The skin may actually feel sweaty or moist although it is no longer sweating. It can also be pale, bluish, and cold when the blood flow to the skin is greatly reduced.

Rapid first-aid treatment is essential for heat-stroke victims. As with heat exhaustion, the victim should be taken to a cool, shady spot as soon as possible and should be made to lie down on one side. This position is especially important if the person feels nauseated or is vomiting. Loosen or remove the person's clothing and, if possible, douse or spray the person with cold water. If you use very cold water or ice, you should also massage the skin in order to counteract the contraction of blood vessels that these cold materials will produce. If the victim is conscious, he or she should drink large quantities of cold water. Hospitalization may be necessary, especially in cases in which the victim is unconscious.

Obviously, heat exhaustion and heat-stroke are dangerous conditions. In order to avoid them, it is important to remember that there is a considerable difference in the amount of heat that different persons can tolerate. Experience also shows that the risk of heat stress can be minimized by following certain guidelines.

GUIDELINES FOR HOT-WEATHER RUNNING AND RACING

Do wear light-colored, lightweight, loose-fitting clothing.
Do drink plenty of water before a run or race.
Do drink frequently during a run or race.
Do douse your body—including your head—with water during a run or race.
Do schedule training runs early in the day.
Do not wear tight clothing.
Do not tuck in your shirt.
Do not wait until you are thirsty before drinking water.
Do not aim for a personal record in a hot-weather race.
Do not run at your top speed.
Do not schedule a longer-than-usual run.
Do not run if you have a fever, flu, or cold.
Do not ignore the symptoms of heat stress.

KEEPING WARM.

In the winter of 1980, a young woman in the frozen Midwest was rushed to the emergency room of a hospital. Her body was frozen solid. Her car had broken down and she had attempted to walk to find help. She had come within steps of a house but had been unable to reach the door, and was found the next morning. Seemingly miraculously, she was revived by doctors and suffered only the loss of a toe. Cold weather can have drastic consequences.

The body loses heat when the temperature of the skin surface is higher than that of the air around it. Our skin temperature is regulated mainly by the circulation of blood in the outer layer of our skin. When we are exposed to the cold, this blood flow decreases, and the skin temperature decreases with it, reducing the loss of body heat because the difference between the skin temperature and the air temperature is reduced. In this way the body protects its more sensitive internal organs against losing heat. In addition, the body uses "shivering" as a mechanism for producing significant amounts of heat.

The combination of cold, wind, and rain can cause rapid heat loss. Most of us have felt the cold biting into our faces when the wind blows, even though the thermometer is only a few degrees below freezing. This is the wind-chill factor. The same temperature in still air can actually feel quite comfortable. The wind makes it especially difficult to maintain the protective layer of air between our skin and the fibers of clothing nearest to it, which is what insulates our bodies against heat loss in cold weather.

As in hot-weather running, being properly dressed applies to training in the winter months. We must protect ourselves from losing too much heat, which can affect performance and lead to a number of injuries including frostbite and hypothermia.

GUIDELINES FOR COLD-WEATHER RUNNING AND RACING

Do wear several layers of clothing: a soft inner layer, absorbent middle layer, and wind-breaking outer layer.

Do wear tights and extra protection for the groin (men especially).

Do wear a warm hat and, if necessary, a balaklava or other face protector.

Do wear layered hand protection—old socks over gloves or mittens, for example.

Do not wear shoes that are snug. Cramped toes mean poor circulation and heat loss.

Do not ignore symptoms of frostbite: small white or yellow-white spots on the skin, and stiffness and numbness. Warm the affected area, such as by placing your hands under your arms.

Do not rub your eyes. Blink instead, to protect the cornea from abrasion.

Do not train hard in very cold (5° F, or -15° C and below) weather.

Do not race if you experience asthma-like symptoms in the cold.

A WORD FOR WOMEN RUNNERS.

In the 1984 Los Angeles Olympics, for the first time in Olympic history, women will participate in the marathon distance. This is a milestone in the effort to bring equality to the sports arena. For many years, Olympic regulations have kept women from competing in the longer distances. It was not until 1972 that there was a 1,500 meter race for women in the Olympic games.

Increasing numbers of women are taking sports as seriously as men do, and participating in races and competitions. People no longer turn their heads when they see a female athlete, whether she is jogging on local streets and pathways or behind the oars in a rowing competition. Yet there are still women who do not participate in any sports or exercise programs. They may believe that hard physical training leads to oversized muscles and a masculine appearance, or they may feel that such activity is not feminine. However, strong muscles are not necessarily large muscles. Most of the top female runners are proof of this. Their training most often leads to long, lithe muscles.

Some women avoid competition because they dislike running in "mixed company." For them, there are many races open only to women. One such race is the annual L'Eggs Mini-Marathon in Central Park in New York City. In 1982, nearly 6,000 women of all ages showed up at the starting line of this 10-kilometer race. For many female runners, these women-only races are truly inspirational.

Women who have been inactive for years should begin to train and to race at a very slow, gradual pace. Most will probably rarely experience any problems; only at the elite level is there the possibility of such difficulties as menstrual irregularity. And these usually disappear when training schedules are relaxed.

The competitive running programs we have outlined may not appeal to everyone. Some readers will be content with their daily exercise regimen and will feel that they have enough pressure in their daily lives without adding the stress of competition in their free time. Others, however, will enjoy the challenge of racing. Their success is not necessarily measured in terms of other runners but of their own goals and expectations for almost every runner has set an individual goal, and how it is reached will determine whether that runner wins his or her race. Thus, every race is really many races. Obviously, there is the race to see who comes in first overall, but there are also the other race categories according to age and sex, and some races include special categories such as the first wheelchair competitor, the first hometown runner, the first lawyer or doctor. And these are only the most visible race results.

A tremendous sense of achievement can be gained by setting and meeting reasonable goals. Pacing yourself in a race is also a way to learn self-control, and the steady training for competition reinforces the habit of self-discipline. As we have discussed throughout this book, these are all factors that will help you control and alleviate the stress in your life.

Selected Reading

This abbreviated list, by no means a complete survey of the vast literature of health and fitness, will give the interested reader a start in exploring in greater depth some of the topics covered in this book.

Aegerter, Ernest. *Save Your Heart*. New York: Van Nostrand Reinhold, 1981.

Benson, Herbert. *The Relaxation Response*. New York: William Morrow, 1975.

Bogert, L. Jean, et al. *Nutrition and Physical Fitness*. Philadelphia: W.B. Saunders, 1973.

Brody, Jane E. *Jane Brody's Nutrition Book*. New York: W. W. Norton, 1981.

Budd, Brian, and Val Clery. *Executive Guide to Fitness*. New York: Van Nostrand Reinhold, 1982.

Carr, Rachel. *Yoga for All Ages*. New York: Simon and Schuster, 1972.

Cooper, Kenneth H. *The New Aerobics*. New York: Bantam Books, 1970.

— *The Aerobics Way*. New York: Bantam Books, 1977.

— and Mildred Cooper. *Aerobics for Women*. New York: Bantam Books, 1972.

Fixx, James. *The Complete Book of Running*. New York: Random House, 1977.

Friedman, Meyer, and Ray H. Rosenman. *Type A Behavior and Your Heart*. New York: Alfred A. Knopf, 1974.

Glover, Bob, and Jack Shepherd. *The Runner's Handbook*. New York: Penguin Books, 1978.

Henderson, Joe. *Run Gently, Run Long*. Mountain View, California: World Publications, 1974.

Hoyt, Creig, et al. *Food for Fitness*. Mountain View, California: World Publications, 1975.

Jackson, Ian. *Yoga and the Athlete*. Mountain View, California: World Publications, 1975.

Kraus, Hans. *Backache, Stress, and Tension*. New York: Simon and Schuster, 1965.

Lance, Kathryn. *Running for Health and Beauty: A Complete Guide for Women*. New York: Bobbs-Merrill, 1977.

Martin, Alice A., and Frances Tenenbaum. *Diet Against Disease: A New Plan for Safe and Healthy Eating*. New York: Penguin Books, 1982.

Mayer, Jean. *A Diet for Living*. New York: David McKay, 1975.

Morella, Joseph J., and Richard J. Turchetti. *Nutrition and the Athlete*. New York: Van Nostrand Reinhold, 1982.

Polunin, Miriam, ed. *The Health and Fitness Handbook*. New York: Van Nostrand Reinhold, 1982.

Selye, Hans. *The Stress of Life*. New York: McGraw-Hill, 1978.

— *Stress without Distress*. New York: J. B. Lippincott, 1974.

Ullyot, Joan L. *Running Free: A Guide for Women Runners and Their Friends*. New York: G. P. Putnam's Sons, 1980.

Verney, Peter. *The Weekend Athlete's Fitness Guide*. New York: Van Nostrand Reinhold, 1982.

Index

Acceptance, 30–31
Achievement anxiety, 66–68
Action paralysis, 39–40
Aging, 106–9
Alcohol, 87
Angina pectoris, 46–47
Anxiety. *See* Nervousness
Atherosclerosis, 46–47
Attitude, 29–30

Bran, 82
Breathing, shallow, 54–56

Carbohydrate, 80, 81
    loading, before racing, 123–25
Cheese, 82
Cigarettes. *See* Smoking
Compensation, 27
Conflict phobia, 41

Defense mechanisms, 25–27
Diet, 80–83
Dietary supplements, 83
Digestive system, 58–59
Distance, from stress source, 32–33
Dizziness, 57
D'Orlando, Maria, 107

Emotional needs, 78–79
Exercise. *See also* Racing
    after age fifty, 106–9
    benefits of, 91
    3-Phase Program, 99–106
    and weight loss, 109–12
Extremities, cold, 52–54

Fat, 80, 81, 82
Fatigue. *See* Weariness
Fiber, 81, 82
Fight-or-flight syndrome, 2
Fish, 82
Fruit, 82

Goals. *See also* Achievement anxiety
    simple, 31–32
    too-high, 27–28
    too many, 28
Guilt, 75–76

Headache, 52
Heart attack, 46, 47
Heart disease, 45–48
Heat exhaustion, 126–27
Heat-stroke, 127
Hill, Ron, 107

Hippocrates, 90
Humor, 27, 29
Hypertension, 48–50

Identification, 26
Impotence, 63–65
Insecurity. *See* Uncertainty
Insomnia. *See* Sleeplessness
Irritation
    as cause of stress, 28–29
    as result of stress, 36–37
Isolation, social, 43

Jogging. *See* Exercise

Lewis, Larry, 107

Menstruation, 60–63
Mental Training Program
    advancing in, 11
    and applied training, 13–14
    Basic Training Sequence #1, 10
    Basic Training Sequence #2, 10
    Basic Training Sequence #3, 12
    Basic Training Sequence #4, 14
    benefits of, 20–24
    and concentration exercises, 12
    deep relaxation during, 11–12
    precautions for, 18–19
    preparation for, 8
    reactions to, 17–18
    theory behind, 5–7
    tips for, 15–20
Milk, 82
Minerals, 80–81
Mueller, Fritz, 107
Muscle tension, 50–52

Nausea, 57
Nervousness, 36
New York Marathon, 107, 113
Nutrition. *See* Diet

Openness, 30
Overstimulation, 68–70

Passivity. *See* Withdrawal
Performance, reduced, 38–39
Phobias, 43–44
PMS (premenstrual syndrome), 60–63
Procrastination. *See* Action paralysis
Protein, 80, 81
Pulse rate, 95–99

Racing
    cold-weather, 128–30
    diet for, 123–26
    hot-weather, 126–28
    training
        competitive, 117
        for occasional racers, 116
        interval, 114–16
        long, slow distance, 114
        marathon, 119–20
        schedules for, 116–20
        ten-kilometer, 117–18
    warm up for, 120–23
    and women, 130–31
Rationalization, 26
Restlessness, 37
Reverse reaction, 26
Role playing, 76–78
Romazzini, 90
Roughage. *See* Fiber

Self-centeredness, 41–42
Self-inflicted pressure, 71–72
Simplicity, 31–32
Sleeplessness, 59–60
Smoking, 83–87
Spontaneity, lack of. *See* Withdrawal
Step test, 91–95
Stimulants, 88–89
Stress. *See also* specific physical and
  mental responses; specific causes
    coping with. *See* Mental Training
      Program
    frequency of, 3
    gearing down after, 4
    intensity of, 3–4
    negative cycle of, 4

physical reaction to, 1–2
purpose of, 2–3
reason for, 1
Suppression, 2, 26–27

Tolerance. *See* Acceptance, 30–31
Tranquilizers, 88–89

Ulcer, 58–59
Uncertainty, 72–74
Understimulation, 68–70

Van Alpen, Piet, 107
Vang, Georg B., 107
Vegetables, 82
Vitamins, 80–81, 82

Water, 81
Weariness, 37–38
Weight loss, 109–112
Withdrawal, 27, 42
Worry, 74